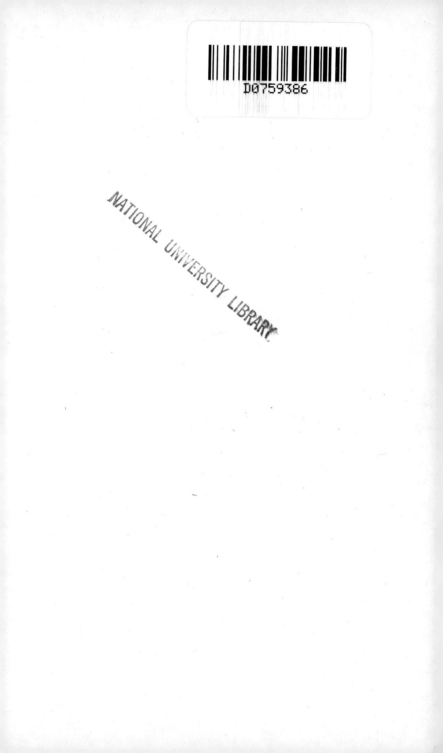

*Methods of Childbirth*

Constance A. Bean

# METHODS OF CHILDBIRTH

NEW, REVISED EDITION

ILLUSTRATED BY PHILLIP JONES

Dolphin Books
Doubleday & Company, Inc.
Garden City, New York
1982

Library of Congress Cataloging in Publication Data
Bean, Constance A.
Methods of Childbirth.
Bibliography: p. 238
Includes index.
1. Childbirth.   2. Prenatal care.   I. Title.
RG525.B42   1982      618.4
ISBN 0-385-17656-2    AACR2
Library of Congress Catalog Card Number 81–43405

BOOK DESIGN BY BENTE HAMANN

# Contents

# Foreword

Over the past two decades, the practice of obstetrics has seen a complete metamorphosis. Where once "twilight sleep" and heavy medication were the norm, now natural, or prepared, childbirth has become increasingly popular. Today, husband participation is considered a necessity and is no longer questioned. Family participation is becoming more accepted as its benefits are realized. Alternative birthing centers and birthing rooms are now a part of every maternity unit. The need for midwives is becoming apparent, and their acceptance by obstetricians is slowly occurring.

The result of all this change has been most beneficial. Modern medical technology, which is being used in the many phases of childbirth, requires the patient's understanding and cooperation, and its use is possible only if the patient is awake and aware.

Similarly, the reduction of maternal mortality and trauma in childbirth has been achieved by a better understanding of the labor process and by the ability of the patient to relax and cooperate with her labor coach.

Natural childbirth proponents claim also that better family relationships and personality adjustment will in the future result from these methods.

Not enough praise and appreciation can be given to such pioneers as Connie Bean and others who have worked so enthusiastically and fervently to spread the gospel of prepared childbirth techniques through their classes and writings. Having experienced the beneficial effects of these methods, they have continued through many adversities until today the results have become evident by nearly everyone in the field. Now they should look back and feel proud that they were a part of this movement.

As Mrs. Bean has stated to me, the purpose of her book is to raise the consciousness of parents and professionals regarding the interrelationship of obstetrical interventions and also the options now available for childbirth.

The book thoroughly explains nearly all hospital procedures and explores how these techniques with their obvious potential benefits can affect the childbirth experience.

Nearly every subject relating to present-day obstetrics, including labor, delivery, methods of preparing for childbirth, breastfeeding, home birth, Cesarean section, and many other topics, are discussed in detail and with such clarity as to make this a most useful book—one that is a must for everyone interested in childbirth.

*Gerald Cohen, M.D., A.C.O.G.*
*Clinical Instructor, Obstetrics and Gynecology*
*Boston University College of Medicine*
*University of Massachusetts College of Medicine*
*Board of Directors*
  *La Leche League*
  *BACE*
  *C-Section*
*Elected Chief of Obstetrics and Gynecology, Leonard Morse Hospital*

# Introduction

"We go to prenatal appointments. My husband will be there for delivery, but we don't know what to expect or even what questions to ask about birth, hospitals, and medical care." This comment, from a pregnant woman, is typical. Natural, or prepared, childbirth is now the rule rather than the exception, and while it has resulted in an improved childbirth experience for parents, it has also opened up a potentially confusing array of options.

Although parents-to-be can seek information from hospitals, consumer health organizations, childbirth educators, and "discussion only" appointments with physicians or midwives, the answers they get may be varied—even conflicting. And, valuable as they are, most childbirth classes just don't have time to address all of an expectant couple's concerns. Typically, the classes don't even begin until the seventh month of pregnancy so that the newly learned Lamaze techniques will be fresh in the couples' minds for delivery. Where do couples go with their questions before that?

The purpose of this book is to provide practical information so that expectant parents can plan their child's birth with knowledge of *all* the options available. This book will examine the bodily processes of pregnancy, labor, and delivery, and will discuss the various methods of preparing for the birth, including those of Lamaze, Bradley, Dick-Read, Kitzinger, and others. Various hospital procedures routinely performed during labor and delivery, as well as after the birth, will be examined showing the advantages and (mostly) the disadvantages of the current technology. Cesarean birth and how to prepare for it, home birth, and alternative birth centers, and patients' rights issues will also be presented in depth.

Although this book will point out emphatically that your doctor doesn't always know what is best for you, and although it will discuss the possible areas of tension between you and medical professionals, its purpose is not to encourage an adversary relationship between consumers and providers of obstetrical care. Rather, this book is meant to give you the information you need to decide how your baby will be born and how you can begin a meaningful dialogue with your doctor and hospital. It is only through such a dialogue that you can ensure that your childbirth experience is as joyful and safe as you want it to be.

# Chapter One

# PREGNANCY, LABOR, AND DELIVERY— WHAT TO EXPECT

"Where do babies come from?" is one of the earliest questions of childhood. However, an entire life may pass without this question being truly answered. Those who wondered as children how babies got born have, until natural childbirth became the norm, frequently grown up and themselves become parents without any first-hand knowledge of the fascinating and universal event of birth. Lack of information about normal reproductive processes can increase your feelings of vulnerability and fear when planning for a birth. Knowing what to expect and learning childbirth skills in a supportive environment, on the other hand, can greatly enrich the experience.

## PREGNANCY

Labor and delivery occur after approximately nine months of pregnancy—actually ten lunar months, or forty weeks. The day of birth is likely to occur within two weeks before or after the so-called due date, or EDC (quaintly, the "expected date of confinement"). The experience of pregnancy is an ever-changing one as the baby grows and the uterus enlarges.

### Conception and Early Development

At ovulation each month an egg leaves one of the two ovaries. The Fallopian tube, not attached to the ovary, has a cupped end that moves to scoop up the emerging egg. The cilia, hairlike structures inside the tube, wave like a field of wheat, their motion carrying the egg toward the uterus. The journey takes about three days. Fertilization, if it occurs, takes place usually in the outer third of the Fallopian tube, before the egg enters the uterus. The first of millions of the male's sperm cells to reach the egg contributes one half of the chromosomes of the new individual, while the female's egg contributes the other half of the total forty-eight chromosomes.

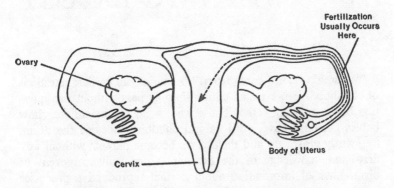

*The uterus, ovaries, and Fallopian tubes*

Almost immediately the fertilized cell begins to divide into more cells on its way to the uterus. After reaching the uterus it floats freely for several days, but about a week after conception it must implant in the soft tissue of the uterus to tap nutrients from the maternal bloodstream. The placenta, or afterbirth, is formed by the fetal structure and attaches to the uterus. It extrudes fingerlike projections into the uterine wall, through which oxygen and nutrients are supplied to the developing baby and through which carbon dioxide and other waste products are carried from the fetus into the mother's bloodstream. The baby's blood and the mother's blood do not mix—in fact, mother and baby may even be of different blood types. Bacteria do not permeate the placental barrier, but viruses, drugs, and certain other substances do pass through.

During these early weeks, when the mother may not even realize that she is pregnant, the infant is most vulnerable to environmental factors such as radiation, drugs, and toxic substances of all types. Even an occasional drink of low alcohol content has been shown by research at the Eunice Kennedy Shriver Center to add significant risk to the fetus. Similarly, smoking during pregnancy has long been known to retard growth and adversely affect fetal brain cells. Now, even the effects of second-hand smoke, as with a cigarette- or pipe-smoking spouse, are also suspected of harm. Tetracycline, a commonly prescribed medication, may retard bone growth.

## The First Trimester

During the first three months, often called the first trimester, menstruation ceases. Other signs of pregnancy may be increased need for sleep and often nausea, both of which may begin at six weeks or even sooner. The extreme fatigue, and especially the nausea, usually disappear quite suddenly after three months of pregnancy. Some women have no such symptoms.

Women often find their own ways of eating to relieve nausea, which may occur in the morning or at any time. No one knows the reason for nausea, but it is believed to result from altered body chemistry. Small, frequent, non-greasy meals that have little odor usually help. Tea and crackers are often suggested, but they contain virtually no nutrients (unless the crackers are made from whole grains and the tea contains milk). Fresh fruits, cold and unsugared, cold chicken, and some cheeses may taste better than some other foods. Vitamin B6 and other B vitamins may help. An empty stomach or a lack of fluids may actually increase nausea.

Many women no longer are willing to take antinausea drugs. Often they are ineffective or produce drowsiness. No drug has been proven safe during pregnancy. Bendectin, which has been used widely in recent years (and also contains vitamin B6) has been associated with increased risk of birth defects. Many women prefer to take B6, increase their fluid intake, and omit the drug.

Also during the first trimester there will probably be weight gain, even though caloric intake may be less than normal because of the initial lack of appetite. Breast changes may occur. These include some enlargement, tenderness, and deepening of the color of the nipples and surrounding areola. Waist measurement may increase, partly because the rib cage begins to enlarge.

An occasional walk in the fresh air may be all the exercise the woman desires at this point, or she may wish to continue a reasonable degree of the exercise she was previously doing. The most important exercise is good posture. She should back up against the wall, tilting her pelvis to flatten her back against the wall while continuing to breathe. She should practice maintaining this position while walking.

Feelings of ambivalence, even for a desired pregnancy, are typical. The commitment to parenthood has been made. Yet, doubts occur about whether this is the time to be pregnant or whether the couple should have waited, especially if she is experiencing fatigue and nausea. Relationships with the spouse and family become especially relevant; also future career plans. There are often increased feelings of vulnerability and dependency. These doubts usually tend to disappear after the first three months when the baby becomes more real and the mother experiences the feelings of well-being typical of the second trimester.

The possibility of miscarriage is greatest in the first trimester (one in five), and a miscarriage can be upsetting whatever the parents' concept of the reason, which is usually unknown. If they feel that it was because of lack of care on their part, the parents will be distressed. If they are told that the fetus was probably defective, they may feel no better because this implies a defect in their reproductive capacity.

Good nutrition is important even though the fetus is still very small. All the body systems are formed during the first fifty-six days of pregnancy. As mentioned elsewhere, alcohol and tobacco should be avoided. Also, the caffeine present in coffee, tea, chocolate, and cola drinks has been linked to an increased risk of birth defects. All non-essential medications should be avoided.

The changes in the baby during the first three months are phenomenal. At one month the embryo is a sixth of an inch long with a rounded body, trunk, and umbilical cord. There is a spine with vertebrae, and the nervous system is beginning to form. The baby develops from the head downward. The facial structures are forming, also the ribs. By six weeks the baby is one-half inch long, with short arms and legs, floating in the amniotic sac and moored by the umbilical cord. The head is bent forward. The heart is a curved tube, and a simple circulatory system has formed, much of it outside the body, including the placenta. The skin is translucent, and internal organs, including the vertebral arteries, can be seen.

At the end of two months, the heart has already been beating for a month. The muscles are beginning to exercise. The skull bones are growing, but some openings between them will still be present at birth. The eyes, previously open, are beginning to close.

During the third month, the baby's growth is rapid. Also at this time, the placenta takes over the additional function of producing female hormones, which, in addition to those supplied by the ovaries, help to maintain the pregnancy.

The first small hairs on the body form at the beginning of the third month. The downy hair all over the body is nearly all shed at the time of birth except for the coarser hair on the baby's crown. The baby swallows the body hair along with the amniotic fluid, which the baby at times drinks during pregnancy.

## Second Trimester

At four months, the baby is six inches long, and the arms and hands are fully shaped but small. The face is narrow with a tiny chin. The eyelids of the closed eyes bulge. Cartilage in the skeleton is turning to bone. The deciduous teeth, which began to form at six weeks, begin to calcify at four months. Also at four months the permanent teeth begin to develop with calcification starting at approximately the time of birth.

By four and a half months of pregnancy thumb-sucking has begun, and by five and a half months the fingernails have reached the fingertips. The baby, now twelve inches long, often grips its cord. The kicking is very noticeable at five months, although the first gentle kicks can be felt before this time.

For the mother, the second trimester of pregnancy is typically a time of increased energy and interest in the baby. Both parents listen to the baby's heartbeat during prenatal visits. Parents read about childbirth and select a childbirth class. They will read about and discuss breast-feeding and parenting in general.

Weight gain picks up, and women often fear, erroneously, that this rate will continue during the rest of the nine months. The mother's blood volume and metabolic rate increase. She should eat well, including each day at least four servings of vegetables, a salad, at least two fruits, including two servings of citrus fruit per day, an egg, milk or milk products, such as yogurt or cheese, and, at each meal, a high-protein food such as meat, fish, chicken, or combination of vegetable proteins or vegetable- and dairy-product protein. Whole-grain bread or cereal is also needed every day. Obstetricians regularly prescribe a vitamin supplement. Some women also like to take some extra vitamins C and E and will also avoid food dyes and additives as much as possible. Soft drinks are avoided because they are non-nutrients and contain sugar or sugar-substitutes, dyes, and often caffeine.

The Recommended Daily Allowance of nutrients as listed by the Federal Government suggests an extra 300 calories per day for the pregnant woman. This is minimum. Many experts feel that an extra 500 calories each day are preferable and, of course, these should not be obtained from so-called junk foods. A rule-of-thumb is to select fresh foods as opposed to packaged and prepared ones.

Questions about the second trimester may include how to prevent "stretch marks" and varicose veins; also hemorrhoids, which are rectal varicose veins. These are by no means an inevitable part of pregnancy. Some feel that this tendency is inherited. Others feel that preventive measures can be taken. Overstretched skin, possibly resulting in reddish lines fading later to white, called stretch marks, can be minimized by avoiding sudden weight or fluid gain, often the result of a binge of highly sugared "junk" foods. Also, correct posture will prevent the swayed back and protruding abdominal muscles that allow the baby to rest against the abdomen instead of resting within the pelvic basin.

Circulation in the legs is improved by avoiding prolonged standing or sitting and, instead, walking, swimming, or bicycling regularly. Lying on the floor with the legs resting on a chair for several minutes two or three times a day aids the return of venous blood. If the veins do swell, they may return to normal after delivery. Poor nutrition may also be a factor in both vein problems and stretch marks.

From the seventh to ninth month the baby grows from thirteen to a length of twenty inches. Fatty tissue is laid down under the skin. The baby's eyes have opened. The baby can both see and hear, and will startle at sudden noises. The baby has periods of sleep and waking, also makes frequent respiratory movements. There is less fluid surrounding the infant, and therefore the baby feels every movement the mother makes. If she lies on her back, the baby may become more active, probably to avoid lying on her bony spine.

At this time, some women feel the baby's feet under their ribs and against the stomach, and they may have to eat smaller meals. They may have some heartburn. Relieving backache involves doing pelvic tilt exercises both on all fours and against the wall (see Chapter Two), also sleeping in a side position.

Hemorrhoids may be prevented by avoiding prolonged sitting or standing and by doing the Kegel exercise in Chapter Two to promote circulation of blood and to strengthen the sphincter muscles around the vagina which are supporting the weight of the growing baby. This exercise will also be done after birth to promote muscle tone of the pelvic floor.

The uterus will probably, during the last month or so, contract noticeably at times (Braxton Hicks contraction) in preparation for the approaching birth. Sometimes muscles and ligaments in the abdomen may give an occasional twinge. Women frequently ask about this, but if this sensation is noticed at times, it is not significant.

Fluid accumulates, often noticeably, in the feet and wrists, especially in hot weather. Extra fluid, unless extreme, is a normal part of pregnancy. Physicians and midwives check this at prenatal visits. The use of diuretics to prevent this normal fluid retention is considered hazardous because blood circulation to the placenta may be diminished.

Women usually can continue working at their jobs until delivery, depending on work conditions. Those working with environmental hazards such as lead, mercury, pesticides, herbicides, dry cleaning and photography chemicals, dusts, X-ray equipment, and many others will want to stop working when pregnancy begins, or even before. Information on these may be obtained from one of the regional offices of the Environmental Protection Agency, as well as from environmental organizations. Those who must stand or remain relatively immobile at the workplace will need to make some kind of change. There are indications that a pregnant woman should not use hot tubs and saunas because blood may be brought to the surface of the body in an effort to regulate body temperature, thus diminishing blood flow to the uterus.

Reasonable exercise should continue during all of pregnancy to maintain cardiovascular fitness. Some obstetricians feel that sudden strenuous or prolonged exercise can result in less oxygen available for the baby. If the mother has maintained good physical condition, has gained 25–30 pounds—for some women 35 pounds—and is in general good health, this not likely to be a concern.

During the last months of pregnancy some women notice a sticky substance on the nipples. This is the colostrum preceding the coming of the milk which will be available to the baby at birth. However, don't be concerned if this does not occur, as it has no correlation with milk supply after birth. Often at this time hormonal changes will increase vaginal lubrication. Mucous membranes in the nose may also swell temporarily.

During the last two to six weeks before the birth of a first baby, the settling of the baby into the pelvis, called "dropping" or "lightening," allows more comfort for the mother. An extra spurt of energy is typical, but often needs to be restrained for both parents. Women who stop work a few weeks before birth often take a daily nap. Those who have a young child nap with the child. Husbands may relax or doze during early evenings at home, since if labor should start during the night, they will want to feel as fresh as possible for the experience of labor and birth.

During the months of pregnancy, it is important for both parents to acknowledge the wide range of feelings, from elation to dismay and doubts about coping, they will face. Communication with each other and a network of supportive people are essential. Careful planning for the birth is an investment that can pay big dividends.

## The Uterus

The uterus is primarily a hollow muscle. When there is no pregnancy, it is about the size of a pear with a capacity of little more than a teaspoon of fluid. During pregnancy, it expands to about the size of a small watermelon. This remarkable expansion in itself generates no pain, although some discomfort may be caused by the pull on ligaments supporting the uterus. The lining of the uterus is rich in blood vessels. During the second two weeks of the menstrual cycle, after the release of the egg from the ovary at ovulation, the lining is especially luxuriant.

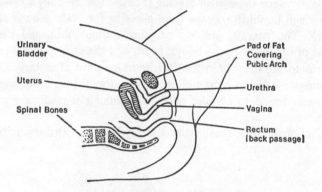

*The pelvic structures*

During pregnancy, the baby is enclosed in the amniotic sac (bag of waters) filled with fluid. The bag of waters, the umbilical cord, and placenta all develop from the fertilized egg, not from the pregnant woman's body. The sac usually breaks sometime during labor. Occasionally, it is the first sign of labor.

Bladder capacity is reduced beginning in the first trimester of pregnancy as the uterus begins its expansion. Frequent urination is less evident during the second trimester, when the uterus rises up and off the bladder, but returns during the last trimester as the uterus all but fills the abdomen and the bladder can hold only a few teaspoonfuls of urine. During labor, an unemptied bladder can produce pain, which is often misinterpreted as labor pain.

## The Vagina

The vaginal tissues, under the influence of the hormone relaxin, soften and expand during late pregnancy, a reassuring piece of information for those who find it hard to believe that a baby can actually fit though that small space. During delivery, the vaginal ridges, called rugae, allow the walls of the vagina to expand to accommodate the approximately four-inch diameter of the baby's descending head. The baby's body ordinarily requires less space than the head since the body has more cartilage and is therefore more flexible. The bones of the baby's head have spaces, or fontanels, between them, also making it easier for the baby's head to fit through the birth passage (and allowing for brain growth after birth). The overall, uniform pressure during labor and delivery is not harmful to the baby's head, and the shape of the head returns to normal within the few hours or days after birth. The compression of the baby's chest as it passes through the vagina has been found to aid the baby in breathing immediately after birth.

After birth, the vaginal tissues quickly lose this extra elasticity.

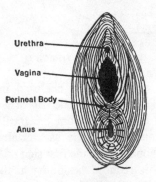

Urethra

Vagina

Perineal Body

Anus

*The vagina, urethra, and anus*

## The Cervix

The cervix is the mouth of the uterus. Normally the opening is no wider than a pencil lead, and it feels firm to the touch, like the ends of two fingers or the tip of one's nose. However, during late pregnancy and labor, hormonal action softens it until it becomes difficult to locate. During childbirth, it opens and pulls over the baby's head in the manner of a turtleneck sweater. The cervix contains few nerves, with the result that the woman cannot feel these changes as it dilates (opens) and effaces (flattens).

## The Pelvis

The pelvic structure forms a bony bowl with an opening in the bottom as well as the top. The lower five vertebrae are fused one to the other culminating in the tailbone. The pubic bones come together in front in a fixed, normally immobile joint. During late pregnancy, this joint softens, and the pelvis expands to create an extra half inch or so of space. This change is often heralded by some pain in this front joint, as well as the tendency to waddle like a duck. The tailbone is less rigid and moves somewhat backward during this time. Even the rib cage expands slightly during pregnancy. After the birth, the softened joints return, like the vaginal tissues, to their pre-pregnant state.

# LABOR

## Labor Contractions: What They Are and What They Feel Like

Labor contractions result from the activity of the uterine muscle fibers, which dilate the cervix to allow the baby to pass through the birth canal. With each contraction, the uterus, which is primarily a hollow muscular organ, tends to rise upward toward the abdominal wall. It then falls back between contractions.

For every woman, both labor and delivery contractions last one minute, with few or temporary exceptions. Like an ocean wave, they rise to a peak for thirty seconds, then subside during the following thirty seconds. During most of the labor, the uterus rests for a longer time than it contracts. The interval between contractions is one minute, two minutes, or five minutes, depending on the individual situation and the stage of labor.

By the way, the uterus contracts at times other than during labor, although these contractions are usually unnoticeable. It contracts during orgasm, for instance. Also, during late pregnancy most women become aware of Braxton Hicks contractions, which are referred to as "practice contractions" for labor. These contractions, which may or may not be painful, usually feel like pressure—which is what all contractions are. Sometimes during the Braxton Hicks contractions the abdomen becomes hard like a basketball for thirty seconds or so. As birth approaches, Braxton Hicks contractions become more frequent and more noticeable. Although they have been called "false labor," they may actually be doing some of the work of "true" labor.

The upper portion of the uterus contracts more strongly; the lower part is more passive. During labor this lower end expands as the muscle fibers relax. However, this expansion can be hampered by emotional stress. Uterine muscle, like that of the heart and the digestive system, is not under voluntary control, but, like digestion and pulse rate, can be affected by emotions. If the upper longitudinal muscle fibers must overcome unusual resistance by the lower circular fibers, labor pain can be intensified.

As the uterus contracts, the baby's head moves deeper into the pelvis, and the longitudinal fibers tend to draw the cervix back up over the baby's head. The lower segment expands like a drawstring purse, maintaining this altered shape even between contractions (although, as we said above, the woman has no sensation of this changed uterine shape). The cervix flattens, and it opens from a diameter about the thickness of the lead of a pencil to about four inches (given in hospital labor records as "five fingers" or "ten centimeters"). The baby's head then passes through the cervix into the vagina.

What do labor contractions feel like? They feel like pressure on muscle (which they are) or like menstrual cramps, except that each lasts just one minute virtually throughout the entire labor. After peaking at the end of thirty seconds, the contraction gradually diminishes for the next thirty seconds. Some women misinterpret the contractions as gas pains or indigestion. Some women whose labors appear to be very short have actually slept through the early hours of labor, reporting that they awakened only enough to change into a more comfortable position. Between contractions, women ordinarily experience no sensations whatsoever, with the possible exception of backache which is not related directly to the contractions. Close to birth, the contractions ordinarily change to the more familiar sensations of rectal pressure, which are usually less anxiety-provoking.

The delivery stage has long been known to be the least painful part of labor. The actual emergence of the baby is not usually felt because of so-called "pressure anesthesia." If the birth is not unusually fast or rushed, the pressure of the baby's head on the vaginal tissues tends to numb them in the same fashion that your foot becomes numb when you sit on it. Usually, the woman has to be told that her baby's head is out if she is not in a position where she can see it for herself.

Intense contractions lasting longer than a minute, which are possible in chemically stimulated labor, may inhibit circulation through the placenta. However, the contractions of a normal labor appear to provide desirable stimulation to the infant. Cesarean babies delivered after labor contractions have begun often fare better after birth than Cesarean babies who have not.

## Labor Pain

The exact source of pain in labor is not known, and the intensity of pain experienced is incredibly varied. Some women report little or none, while others experience strong pain, at least at times, during their labor. The degree of satisfaction women receive from their labor does not seem to be directly related to the amount of pain they experience. Some even report disappointment that it was all over so quickly that they never had a chance to do the breathing they learned in their childbirth classes. Those who have had difficult labors, but who have received adequate training, along with the help and encouragement of their husbands and hospital staff, often take pride in being able to lessen their pain through childbirth education techniques. Some women forego the techniques for one contraction in order to see the difference, which helps to give them a feeling of being in control of the pain they experience.

Those who do feel severe pain should try to discover the reason in the break between contractions; perhaps they will wish to ask their doctors or nurses about a possible medical reason. Many women and men who have given up their traditional fears about childbirth prefer to have solid answers rather than to take the quick recourse to medicated oblivion. Moreover, the perception of pain is influenced by the meaning of that pain. Whether it is a result of normal body functioning during labor or an indicator of a medical problem makes a significant difference to the patient and her mate. In any case, the pain associated with birth is intermittent, has a predictable pattern, a purpose, and a definite end. And each contraction lasts just one minute.

Strong contractions usually mean that the labor is progressing, since weak ones lasting less than sixty seconds are less effective in dilating the cervix. Therefore, there is reason to welcome effective contractions. Also, many aware people are learning that the experience of a "reasonable" degree of pain is not always one they need or wish to avoid. It is a sensation with meaning, but is not necessarily associated with suffering and fear.

Most women prefer the pain of labor contractions to that of common occurrences, such as a severe headache. Labor pain is in no way as severe as that from a dental drill or banging one's shins against a hard object. Kidney stone pain is considered far worse than labor pain, as is angina. Women who have experienced menstrual pain or painful intercourse report no correlation between this and the pain they experience in childbirth, and are often pleasantly surprised.

One theory does suggest that labor pain is caused by a lack of adequate oxygen to the uterine muscles, as the suffering of angina patients is ascribed to a lack of oxygen to the heart muscle. This may be one reason for the effectiveness of the prepared childbirth breathing techniques.

The pain associated with labor contractions may also be relieved by relaxing tight abdominal muscles, which can interfere with the contracting uterus. Also, the woman should *never* lie flat on her back during labor, since this position pulls the abdominal muscles taut against the contracting uterus, causing pain and reducing the blood flow to the uterus, which can reduce the supply of oxygen to the baby.

The pain of delivery can be relieved if the woman assumes a semi-sitting position, or another position that allows the force of gravity to aid the birth. If she were to be flat in the traditional position designed for gynecological surgery, on the other hand, the woman would be pushing the baby uphill, since the vagina is angled downward toward the small of the back. Learning to relax the muscles surrounding the vagina is another way to relieve possible pain, even though pressure anesthesia by itself can be effective.

The importance of encouragement on the part of husband and

medical staff cannot be overemphasized. And since medications are available, a woman need never feel more sensation than she wishes. However, it is necessary to learn about these drugs beforehand to understand their uses and possible side effects. Also, it's not a good idea to take medication out of fear, or for anticipated rather than actual pain, since many anesthetized women later complain that they didn't feel well afterward, or didn't feel in control of their baby's birth. Also, many women report that, ironically, they asked for medication not realizing that the birth was imminent and that their labor was virtually over.

Other techniques for relieving pain in childbirth are discussed in the following chapter.

## The Stages of Labor

There are three stages to every labor.

In the *first stage* of labor, the cervix dilates from its usually tiny opening to a diameter of 5 fingers or 10 centimeters. This is all that happens at this stage. The baby does not yet move from the uterus.

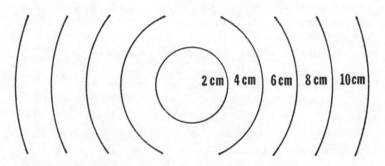

2 cm  4 cm  6 cm  8 cm  10cm

*Dilation of the cervix during the first stage of labor, to "5 fingers," or approximately 10 centimeters. (Shown actual size.)*

The first is the longest stage of labor, although exactly how long is not always easy to define because, as has been stated, the cervix may begin its effacement and dilation before the woman has any awareness of uterine activity. In many instances, the Braxton Hicks contractions of pregnancy will already have done some of the work of early labor. One sign that labor is beginning is the "show," when the protective mucous plug in the cervix becomes dislodged and tiny capillaries break to make the plug pinkish or blood-streaked. Because of the increased amount of vaginal discharge in late pregnancy, the woman may be unaware of the discharged plug unless it is blood-streaked.

The first stage has been known to last for as little as a single observable contraction to on-again-off-again labor over a span of two or three days, or even longer. Eleven to fifteen hours has been described as optimium for a first baby because it is less stressful to both woman and baby than a shorter, harder labor.

Even after labor is obviously established with a regular pattern of contractions two to five minutes apart, accurate predictions about the length of this stage are impossible. At first, the dilation is slow, but afterward it continues at an ever-increasing rate, so that, for example, a dilation of 5 centimeters after eight hours does not indicate that eight more hours will be required for full dilation.

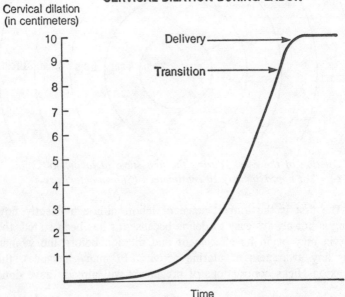

**CERVICAL DILATION DURING LABOR**

Cervical dilation
(in centimeters)

The amniotic sac, or bag of waters, usually breaks sometime during the first stage. In fact, the resulting sudden gush of warm fluid may be the first sign of labor. In other cases, it may not rupture until the expulsion stage. Or the membrane may be broken by the hospital staff shortly after admission to speed the labor. This procedure is discussed in Chapter Five.

*Transition* is not a separate stage of labor, but is really the end of the first stage. In fact, when women were medicated to the point of unconsciousness or hallucination under the amnesic drug Scopolamine, obstetrical texts did not recognize transition as even a separate phase of labor. The process of transition was defined only after women were awake and participating in their labor.

Transition, which occurs between 7 and 10 centimeters of cervical dilation, is the shortest and most uncomfortable part of the labor for most women. For a first baby it can be expected to last a maximum of forty-five minutes, or fifteen contractions, whichever occurs first. For subsequent babies, transition is shorter. Some women do not experience it at all, and after assiduously practicing their comfort techniques for this stage some couples find no need to use them.

The signs of transition are variable, but an observer can usually tell when the woman enters transition because there is a sharp mood change. She can become irritable and uncooperative with no evidence of any interest in the baby. She can become critical of her mate and refuse to let him touch her. She can become apathetic, appearing to be in a state of extreme fatigue. Sometimes there is a premature urge to push as the uterus prepares for the second stage, expulsion. The woman should be informed that she is in transition. Otherwise, feeling that the birth is not going well for her, she may opt without real cause for an anesthetized, forceps birth, only to be furious later because nobody told her that her negative perceptions were due to her arrival at transition, the most difficult part of the birth.

Other signs of transition are irregularly spaced contractions that may also be variable in length instead of the expected sixty seconds they have been and will be again. Often the contractions feel more painful than they did previously. Sometimes, the woman in transition feels very warm and throws off her covers or clothes. Other women begin to shiver with cold. Sometimes her legs shake for no apparent reason. (This may also occur immediately after birth for a minute or two, also for no apparent reason, although the shivering is variously ascribed to emotions or hormonal action.) Occasionally the woman becomes nauseous during transition, and some observers feel that the long period of fasting during labor may produce this symptom, although this is not known for certain. In any case, each woman will experience only one or two of the above symptoms, not all of them. In fact, some women experience none of them and even express a twinge of regret if they haven't felt transition.

Transition usually ends as suddenly as it arrived. The woman feels renewed energy and interest in her surroundings. Often contractions stop for a period of ten minutes or so immediately after transition.

The *second, or expulsive, stage* is usually the most enjoyable for the woman, since after hours of using the relaxation techniques, she can finally take an active role in moving the baby down the birth canal. During this stage, she pushes as hard as the contraction demands with the sphincter muscles of the vagina relaxed. She can hasten birth or slow it as desired. Usually she pushes only with the contraction, but she could push between contractions to hasten birth. Gentle birth and gentle pushing are the current goal for the benefit of both mother and baby.

*The second stage of labor*

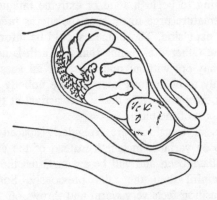

*At the beginning of the second stage, the cervix is fully dilated.*

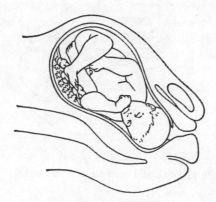

*The uterus, aided by the diaphragm and other respiratory muscles, begins to move the baby down the birth canal.*

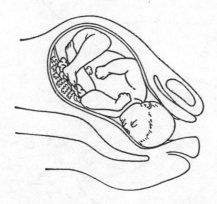

*Each contraction moves the baby closer to birth.*

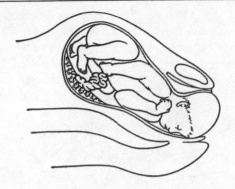

*The baby's head begins to appear during the height of the contraction, but disappears again between contractions.*

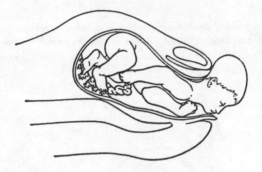

*The crowning*

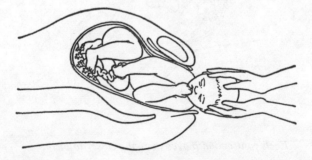

*The baby's head turns to the side as the top shoulder is about to emerge.*

The second-stage contractions occur every two or three minutes and, as before, last for one minute. This expulsive stage may consist of only two or three contractions. More typically, it is one to one-and-a-half hours, or, with the new gentle birth techniques, often two hours or more. During this second stage of labor, the baby is moved down the birth canal by the action of the uterus, aided by the diaphragm and the other respiratory muscles. During pregnancy the baby usually has been lying sideways, not facing the mother's front or back. Often, if the left side of her abdomen protrudes slightly more than the opposite side this means that the baby's back and buttocks are on that side.

During the second stage the cervix slides back over the baby's head and body until, if one could see internally, the uterus and vagina would appear to be one continuous passageway. The baby's head is now turned by both the expulsive forces and the bony structure of the pelvis to face downward.

From outside the mother's body first the vaginal tissues can be seen to quiver during a pushing contraction. Then a small part of the crown of the baby's head may be seen at the height of the contraction. It then disappears. During subsequent contractions more of the baby's head may be seen during the contraction, only to disappear between contractions. The part of the baby seen may appear grayish in color because the baby has not yet breathed. Because the back of the baby's head, the crown, is being seen, the color of the baby's hair, although wet, may be evident. When a substantial part of the baby's head is seen, perhaps two inches, the head can be seen between as well as during contractions. The next contraction will bring the entire crown of the baby's head and the baby's head is then described as having "crowned."

The baby's head may emerge slowly or almost pop out. The baby turns its head to the side to line it up with the rest of the body still inside. There may be a pause of a few seconds before the rest of the body slides out or the entire baby may emerge almost in one contraction. The creamy vernix on the baby's body lubricates the slide into the outside world.

The baby may draw its first breath as soon as the chest is freed, or when the entire baby emerges. There is a pause, the lungs then inflate, and with the first exhalation breath may make a sound or cry as the air passes through the vocal cords.

The newly born infant can be put immediately to the mother's breast for comforting and to stimulate the mother's milk supply. A small amount of yellowish fluid called colostrum, containing protein and antibodies, is available from the mother at birth. Also, the suckling of the baby helps the mother's uterus to contract by stimulating production of the hormone pitocin.

The *third stage* of labor, which usually occurs within five to ten minutes of the delivery, consists of the expulsion of the placenta. After the baby is born, the uterus shrinks to the size of a grapefruit. The placenta, no longer able to adhere to the wall of the shrinking uterus, is squeezed out of the mother's body. Although the parents are not always aware of this stage, because they are usually absorbed by their new baby, the mother may sit up and help to push out the afterbirth. Or, if she is anesthetized the obstetrician may press on her abdomen and reach inside to help remove it. When the placenta delivers spontaneously, it may feel rather like a bowl of pudding as it slips through the vagina. On the other hand, there may be no sensation at all. There may or may not be a perceptible contraction as it is expelled.

The placenta looks like a small, round pie of eight or nine inches in diameter. It is dark red inside the amniotic sac, and its iridescence makes it sparkle when held to the light. (The amniotic sac, by the way, has been found to be useful for covering the tissues of burn victims.)

## The Umbilical Cord

Few people, unless they have been to a childbirth education series or have attended a birth, have a clear picture of how the cord is cut after delivery.

During pregnancy, the cord, which is approximately the thickness of a man's finger, and which can vary in length from sixteen inches to almost three feet, is attached to the placenta, supplying nutrients and oxygen to the baby and removing waste products. At birth, the umbilical cord is a silvery blue, which gradually fades to a pale gray and then to white within a few minutes. At the same time, its characteristic stiffness, which during pregnancy made knotting of the cord unlikely, begins to fade, the cord gradually becomes limp, and the cord pulsations which can be felt at birth, disappear.

Many obstetricians used to clamp the cord immediately after birth, cut it and, with almost one motion hand the baby to a nurse, who placed it in some type of box, either an incubator, crib, or warming unit. More recently, this sequence of events in the first minutes after birth has begun to change, with expediency no longer the goal (see Chapter Six).

## Blood Loss after Birth

The amount of blood the mother loses after birth may be as little as half a cupful. In fact, many birth attendants who assist at home births observe little or almost no maternal bleeding in those surroundings, because the third stage is not hurried and the baby is put immediately to the breast, which helps the uterus to contract. Significantly more blood is usually lost with most forms of anesthesia (see Chapter Three, "Medication and Anesthesia for Childbirth").

Also, the blood is mixed with the remainder of the amniotic fluid, or "hindwaters," which often makes the blood loss appear greater than it actually is. If an episiotomy incision to enlarge the birth opening has been made, there will also be blood from this procedure. Fortunately, the trend is away from routine episiotomy.

After the birth, the mother experiences a heavier-than-usual menstrual period, lasting perhaps two weeks or longer. This flow, which gradually turns from red to brown, then disappears, is called the lochia.

Because the blood loss after the birth is caused by the shedding of uterine tissue no longer needed, it is totally normal and has nothing to do with injury. Rather, since this bleeding is associated with the beginning of a new life, even first-time parents are seldom bothered by it. Instead, almost uniformly, they are awed by the entire experience of birth and by the newborn's responsiveness to sight, sound, and touch. Very often, couples describe the birth of their child as the most beautiful experience of their lives.

## Emergency Childbirth

Sudden births do happen with little warning in places where there is minimum space and it is difficult to be comfortable, such as an automobile. Instead of continuing the frantic dash to the hospital, the husband should stop the car if birth is imminent as evidenced by the mother's feeling of pressure and sense that the baby is "right there." The urge to push may be strong. If the mother feels this before starting for the hospital or birth center, the couple should stay at home.

If the birth does take place in a car, and the back seat is roomy, the husband may help his wife into a semi-reclining or an all-fours position. She may prefer to deliver over the edge of the seat, in which case she can remain in the front seat as long as the steering wheel doesn't impair the husband's ability to assist.

A coat, raincoat, blanket, or towels under the mother helps to prevent soaking the car upholstery with fluid and blood, which is difficult to dry and to clean up. The amniotic fluid by itself is clear and, in fact, sterile. It has no odor except possibly a faintly sweet smell.

The husband next helps the woman to relax as completely as possible. As the baby emerges, he should urge the mother to pant with shallow breaths to prevent pushing. The squeezing action of the uterus provides adequate force, and if she doesn't increase the pressure by active pushing, there is less chance of the external vaginal tissues tearing. Although the mother will not normally feel any tear if it should occur, it will have to be stitched by the obstetrician later at the hospital or his or her office.

During the delivery, the husband supports his baby's head and body as it emerges. Interestingly, traditional delivery tables are designed to end abruptly at the woman's buttocks to allow the physician access to the patient. So even in the delivery room someone must be stationed at the foot of the table to catch the baby.

The husband does not pull on the baby or on the cord. After the baby is born, the mother or father, or both, cradles him or her. The mother should put the baby to her breast, since nursing helps to contract her uterus, as previously explained, by stimulating a hormonal reflex. Also, the ability of the baby to suck reassures the parents that the child is responding normally. The baby must be well wrapped as soon as he or she begins breathing which is usually within a few seconds, or perhaps a little longer. This includes making a hood out of towels or a blanket to prevent heat loss from the baby's head as well as from the rest of the body.

Most babies born away from the hospital breathe very well immediately after birth. Breathing can be aided by massaging the baby's back, legs, and arms, and by flexing them to stimulate breathing reflexes. The baby can even be gently "folded in half" several times to compress the chest. Any mucus in the baby's mouth can be dislodged with a finger, if needed.

The woman and baby should then be taken to an obstetrician or midwife to be examined. However, mother and baby may stay together whether they remain at the hospital or are discharged home. No longer is the litany heard, "The baby was born outside of the delivery suite and is therefore 'contaminated' and must go to the pediatric nursery instead of the newborn nursery." Many hospitals are now agreeable to the parents keeping the baby with them from the moment of birth, and never admit the newborn to a central nursery whether or not the baby is born in the hospital.

## The Baby

The baby does not need to cry after birth, whether born in a hospital or anywhere else. The gentle birth procedures, now available to many parents, often do not elicit the crying "to clear the baby's lungs." The newborn's response to gentle birth is variable. Sometimes the baby simply begins breathing and doesn't make any sound until later, while sometimes, as the air passes through the vocal cords for the first time, the baby makes a sound that cannot quite be described as a cry. Sometimes, even with gentle birth, the baby does cry.

Newborn babies have keen hearing and are easily startled by sudden sounds. They are very responsive to touch—holding, fondling, gentle massage. Contrary to most earlier thought, babies also see at birth (and even before birth, through the abdomen, if the mother stands in a bright light). They see best at a distance of about sixteen inches (which happens to be the distance between the breast and their mother's face). Most adults tend almost instinctively to lean near a new baby's face when talking to him or her. Newborns track objects with their eyes (especially the human face) if their eyes are shielded from bright light. Eye contact between parents and baby has been found to be especially important during the first hour after birth, known as the time of "bonding." Bonding also occurs in the animal world and has been known to psychologists for years. John Kennell, M.D., and Marshall Klaus, M.D., professors of pediatrics at Case Western Reserve Medical School, found bonding to be important in establishing the parent-child relationship and to have long-term effects, as demonstrated by more eye contact and body contact between parent and child during the succeeding months. It is surmised that cognitive development may be enhanced by the opportunities to bond.

After the initial hour, babies tend to withdraw, and their faces become less responsive. They may sleep. If parents could choose just one of the hospital options that are becoming available to them, they would be well advised to avoid the traditional parent-baby separation after delivery and to allow time for bonding with their baby after the birth.

## POSSIBLE MEDICAL PROBLEMS: THE "WHAT IFS"

Many routine childbirth procedures are predicated on the possibility of something going wrong. For years, the public accepted a passive role and depersonalized care with its associated discomforts and inconveniences because of the fear of something "going wrong." Without concrete knowledge, that "something" can only elicit non-specific fears. Actually, problems sometimes come from using procedures designed for high-risk patients on all women, as we will discuss later.

Ivan Illich, in his writings, decries people passing through normal life processes as "patients" because of the politics of medical care. Sometimes there is genuine need for medical treatment, and the mother and baby then do fall in the category of "patients."

But the more modest obstetricians describe themselves as insurance: Although they are normally not needed, they are there in case something goes wrong.

For years, approximately 95 percent of births were considered "normal." However, during the 1970s that figure declined as new categories of patients were defined as high risk: teenage mothers and women over thirty-five (although this classification is controversial in regard to older mothers, it is known that Down's Syndrome, a form of mental retardation formerly known as mongolism, does increase in incidence with the age of the mother). The definition of "high risk" has become politically charged. There are those who wish to define all childbirth as potentially high risk and feel that all available technology should be employed in every birth. "A birth is only normal in retrospect," they say. Because insurance reimbursement mechanisms and other institutional needs can support this stance, the problems of this viewpoint are often circumvented with the rationalization, "At least she got a healthy baby."

Here is a summary of the more likely risk factors and possible complications:

a) Bleeding during pregnancy or labor can indicate a problem. During early pregnancy, some women experience a small amount of bleeding, either spotting or staining. Miscarriage is a possibility here, especially if accompanied by cramps, since approximately one in five conceptions results in miscarriage. Frequently, however, this symptom disappears at the end of the first trimester, and there is no further problem with the pregnancy or birth. Bleeding in later pregnancy is more serious, and may indicate a problem with the attachment of the placenta to the uterine wall. The first sign of approaching labor for many is the "bloody show," as previously described, and this sort of bleeding is quite normal.

On the other hand, substantial bleeding during labor, though very rare, may indicate partial or complete detachment of the placenta (abruptio) or the placement of the placenta over the mouth of the uterus (placenta previa), preventing the birth from occurring. When bleeding occurs from either of these conditions, an emergency Cesarean section must be done. Obstetricians who perform home births state that these problems are virtually the *only* medical emergencies in childbirth where speed is imperative. Whether the woman is in the labor room or ten minutes away from the hospital, an operating team must be ready. Why the placenta detaches in these rare instances is not known. However, an abruptio can be caused, or is assumed to be caused, by pushing hard on the abdomen of an anesthetized woman in order to expel the baby.

Excessive bleeding after birth occurs most often as a result of anesthesia-induced relaxation of the uterus, manual removal of the placenta, or clots in the uterus not expelled after birth. Most experts say that the most serious kind of hemorrhage is slow and prolonged, which gives ample time for blood transfusion. In such a case, intravenous fluids with a drug (Pitocin) to contract the uterus are also started, and the uterus may be held by bimanual compression, with one hand on the abdomen and one hand inside the vagina. Sometimes injections of Pitocin are given; ordinarily, these are effective immediately.

**b)** Cord compression is another rare but serious complication. After the bag of waters is ruptured and there is no amniotic fluid protecting the cord, it is possible for the baby's descending head to compress the cord against the uterine wall and bony pelvis. If the fetal heart rate drops substantially or if the cord can be seen to be coming before the baby, the woman is usually turned onto the knee-chest position and the physician called. For the knee-chest position she gets onto all fours, bending her elbows so that her hips are higher than her shoulders. This may take some pressure off the cord.

If the baby has "dropped" into the pelvis or "lightened," meaning that the baby is down into the pelvis and therefore no longer pressing against the woman's stomach or rib cage, there is little chance of this occurring. A first baby may drop as early as several weeks before birth, while subsequent babies may drop as late as the beginning of labor. If the baby stays high, it may mean that the mother's pelvis is not large enough. In any event, this is a contraindication for any sort of out-of-hospital birth. In earlier days, when induced labor and "babies by appointment" were more common, inductions were sometimes done when the head was still high. The outcome was not always favorable.

c) It's also possible for the cord to become tight around the baby's neck. Usually it is looped loosely around the neck at birth and is unlooped like a necklace at delivery. If it is tight when the head is born, it is quickly clamped and cut so that the baby can breathe.

d) Prematurity is a relatively common problem. This may result for reasons unknown. One known cause is a weak or "incompetent" cervix. Sometimes this is a result of the mother's exposure to DES in utero. Prematurity may also be due to lack of adequate maternal weight gain during pregnancy from undernutrition or malnutrition, or it may be caused by previous uterine surgery. A previous premature baby may increase this possibility for a subsequent baby. Mothers under sixteen years old have an increased chance of having a baby of less than 5½ pounds.

As discussed elsewhere, cigarette smoking and alcohol consumption increase the risk of low birth weight and premature birth.

Medical treatment may be sutures in the prematurely dilating cervix to hold it almost closed as it normally is until late pregnancy. The "circlage," as this procedure is called, will be removed before delivery.

e) The breech position, where the baby comes buttocks down instead of head down, occurs in 2 or 3 percent of births. During pregnancy, the obstetrician or midwife can readily ascertain the position of the baby. If the baby is still breech at the time of delivery, a Cesarean section will most likely be done, since Cesarean birth eliminates the uncertainties associated with manually extracting a baby who may not deliver spontaneously. Obstetricians are no longer being trained to do breech deliveries. However, if the birth is not the woman's first baby, if the pelvis is large enough, if she requests a trial of labor, and if the obstetrician is over forty-five years old and trained to perform breech deliveries, the decision may be for a vaginal birth.

f) Another problem is what is called "the persistent posterior position" where the baby's head is pointing down, but is facing the mother's front, instead of in the usual face-back direction. Many babies start out in this position, and this can usually be ascertained by the obstetrician or midwife, either through an internal vaginal examination or palpation of the abdomen before labor.

If the baby is in the posterior position, there are ways the woman can help to turn it, so that the face points backward. She can walk during labor, sit on the john or in a similar squatting position, or, especially, get up on all fours for much of her labor. Symptoms of the persistent posterior position can be prolonged labor or excessively painful labor, including especially severe back pain.

A persistent posterior baby is a not-infrequent possibility, and may require a forceps birth. Figures as high as 10 percent are given for posterior babies, but for women who do not labor on their backs this figure is probably too high.

g) Prenatal visits during pregnancy can illuminate many potential problems. Elevated blood pressure or urinary test abnormalities require medical attention, as they could—rarely—portend toxemia and a possible need for an induced labor or a Cesarean birth. Toxemia is rare today for reasons not entirely known but the decrease is perhaps associated with increased protein intake and appropriate weight gain.

Anemia is a possibility. Blood tests are done during pregnancy to determine the iron content of the blood. The prenatal diet may be low in other nutrients, but iron deficiency is easily detected by a simple blood test included in all prenatal care.

Rubella, commonly known as German measles, can cause birth defects, especially during the first trimester.

Diabetes in the mother requires close medical supervision all through pregnancy as well as special care for the baby afterward. If the mother is diabetic, the onset of labor is often well beyond the due date, and induction of labor or a Cesarean section may be indicated.

Insufficient weight gain during pregnancy can put both mother and baby at risk for miscarriage, prematurity, low birth weight, maternal fatigue during labor, and slow postpartum recovery. The milk supply of the mother after birth may also be limited.

Obesity during pregnancy has long been considered a hazard for many reasons. The baby's heart may be difficult to hear. The mother's blood pressure is apt to become elevated. If she is trying to control her weight, her diet may be low in essential nutrients and high in sugary junk foods.

Cigarette smoking during pregnancy decreases the baby's oxygen supply and limits fetal growth. As a result, women who smoke are more likely to have low-birth-weight babies and premature babies. Prematurity and low birth weight are the major risks to newborns today.

More recently, maternal consumption of alcohol, even in small amounts, has been found to have observable effects on the baby. These include increased risk of miscarriage, low birth weight, heart defects, mental retardation, a particular pattern of facial deformities, and perhaps others. It is well to note that some over-the-counter cold and sleep remedies contain up to 25 percent alcohol.

The mother's pelvis may be "inadequate," meaning that it is smaller than is required for passage of the baby. Many women can deliver a baby through a so-called "borderline" pelvis if they do not lie on their backs during labor, but walk and do the squatting exercise taught in prepared childbirth classes, especially during the second stage of labor. Because of the ready availability of "safe" Cesareans, careful physical measurements of the pelvis during pregnancy are often neglected. A prolonged labor may indicate such cephalo-pelvic disproportion, or if labor does not progress, this may be assumed to be the cause. Women who ask their physicians during pregnancy about pelvis size often report misleading and vague answers. Doctors often depend on ultrasound pictures, but these cannot tell the whole story, including the size of the baby.

h) Meconium during labor requires careful watching, as it may or may not indicate a problem. Meconium is a black, tarry intestinal material normally excreted by the baby soon after birth. If the amniotic waters are not clear, but brown or green, the fetal heart is checked more carefully during labor and immediately after birth to watch for inhalation of meconium-stained fluid. The relaxation of the baby's anal sphincter during labor instead of after, which causes the meconium to be released early, may have no significance, or it may indicate fetal distress. At birth, there must be care that the baby does not inhale the meconium-stained fluid, or a lung infection may result. Babies with meconium-stained waters are suctioned after birth by using a bulb-suctioning device or more sophisticated equipment (see Chapter Six). These problems are less likely if certain precautions are taken during labor: 1) avoid laboring on the back, which may result in oxygen deprivation for the baby, and 2) avoid unnecessarily induced or speeded labor.

i) Finally, some complications may arise from routine interventions used in many hospitals. For example, the use of the substance Pitocin to stimulate labor may produce fetal distress. Pain medications may slow the labor. Regional anesthesia such as spinals, saddle blocks, and epidurals usually require a forceps delivery and possible catheterization of the mother afterward. Confinement to bed may increase the mother's discomfort and inhibit the progress of labor. Intentionally rupturing the membranes combined with a labor that does not progress may require a Cesarean. An infection for mother or baby occasionally results from the use of fetal heart monitoring equipment, which requires the insertion of electrodes into the fetal scalp inside the uterus. All medications given the mother are now known to pass through the placenta to the baby with various effects on the child. The above medical procedures have become so routine that a detailed look at their advantages and disadvantages will be a major focus of this book (see Chapters Five, Six, and Seven).

# Chapter Two

# METHODS OF CHILDBIRTH

Parents were long intimidated from active participation in childbirth because of its association with sex, surgery, and blood, and because of feelings of inadequacy in the face of the godlike medical profession. The fear of pain, however, was probably the most powerful deterrent. In fact, the primary inducement for middle- and upper-class women in the 1920s to leave their homes and follow the widening stream of charity patients into hospitals for the births of their children was not the promise of improved safety, but the promise of "twilight sleep" and the accompanying freedom from pain.

Not until approximately 1970 were the public and the obstetrical personnel convinced that non-pharmacologic methods of pain relief were effective. Before 1950 only a few women with access to the methods of Dr. Grantly Dick-Read had sought out non-medicated childbirth. In the sixties their numbers increased, but there were years of physician resistance to "allowing" natural childbirth. A frequent admonition was, "Do it the usual way for your first baby, and after you've proved your childbearing capacity maybe you can have natural childbirth next time." Sometimes bewildered women were told, "Natural childbirth is dangerous. Besides, it won't work." It was difficult for parents to buck such advice. Often, in fact, it was more ridicule than advice.

Obstetricians genuinely believed that natural childbirth would not work. They had no reason to believe it would, since they were untrained in natural-childbirth techniques. Also, the new methods prevented them from managing labor and delivery with their accustomed tools, and it appeared to diminish their authority and professional status. It required more discussion and planning with parents-to-be. Patients tended to refuse elective induction of labor (babies by appointment), which had allowed obstetricians to plan their deliveries. ("If we don't start you up on Saturday, I can't promise to be there.") Although there were notable exceptions, many obstetricians hoped that if they disparaged natural childbirth and those who defended it, it would all go away.

Ultimately, obstetricians did recoup their authority over new parents in ways not even imagined in the fifties and sixties, by the emergence of high-technology birth techniques to coexist with obstetrical acceptance of natural childbirth. We will discuss this technology in depth in Chapters Four, Five, Six, and Seven.

## NATURAL CHILDBIRTH

Natural childbirth is better described as "prepared" childbirth, but despite attempts to change its name, many prefer the appellation "natural." By either name, it means informed childbirth, including preparation for and information on birth processes and comfort measures. Little or no medication or anesthesia is anticipated, and if there is a complication, the informed couple participates in the decision resolving the problem.

Prepared childbirth is not defined in terms of "success" or "failure." Medical treatment is used when there is a reason, but parental resentment, anger, and rage, even, can result when expedient intervention replaces time, concern, and encouragement. Natural childbirth assumes the presence of mate or friend, and sometimes the employment of a labor-support person responsible to the couple, not the hospital. At least two persons, including the woman in labor, are needed to work with each contraction.

Childbirth preparation provides information on and practice of comfort techniques, including methods of breathing. Lamaze, Bradley, Kitzinger, or other methods of preparation, all of which have similar effective techniques, may be used. Preparation should also include information on breast-feeding, which like labor and delivery, is a skill to be learned, however natural the process. Just as misinformation and discouragement can alter the rest of the childbirth experience, a few wrong words can end the breast-feeding experience for the couple and baby. Conversely, encouragement and accurate information have resulted in a more joyous birth and breast-feeding experience than the parents would have thought possible.

The varying definitions of natural childbirth can be puzzling. Two couples may ask for natural childbirth, but during labor one woman may be lying awake with an intravenous needle in her arm into which a nearby pump is introducing a labor stimulant. She may be attached to electronic monitoring equipment and may be wearing an oxygen device. A few doors away the second woman, wearing her own clothes, may be sitting in a rocking chair, sipping a glass of cider with none of the above procedures. At her child's birth there will be no gowns or masks, and she will deliver in the same room, the birthing room, instead of being moved to a delivery room. An older sibling might be in the room, too. A third prepared couple on the other hand, may go to Cesarean classes. Both parents may be in the delivery room, and the mother may be awake for the surgery. But despite the obvious preparation and involvement of this couple, no one has yet described a Cesarean as natural childbirth. In other words, by some definitions, all childbirth with the exception of Cesarean section is "natural."

In general, though, most prepared parents expect that, whether or not there is a desire for medication, there will be few or no unnecessary interventions, and that the birth will be spontaneous (that is, not assisted by forceps) unless there is a clear medical need. The couple expects to remain together and to have access to their child at birth and afterward.

# METHODS OF PREPARING FOR CHILDBIRTH

## The Read Method

The first method of relieving labor pain physiologically was developed in the 1940s by the late Dr. Grantly Dick-Read of England. The Read approach, or a modified Read approach, is still used, and the principles on which he based his teaching have continued to stand the test of time. The exercises developed for Read classes by the physical therapists Helen Heardman and Mabel Fitzhugh continue to be effective for childbirth preparation.

The Read method is based on the fear-tension-pain cycle in which fear causes tension which in turn produces pain. Dick-Read stayed with his patients in labor, talked with them, offered information and comfort. Women were taught relaxation and breathing methods. He observed that birth need not be painful. He saw it as beautiful.

Read-based classes have been characterized by more passivity on the part of the woman, more turning inward, more body awareness, than Lamaze classes, which look for ways of distraction from uterine stimuli. Those who prefer the Read approach aim for awareness of all body sensations, and with the help of their partners, select body positions and breathing methods to respond effectively to the sensations of labor. Conscious deep muscle relaxation is recognized as the key to pain relief, and "huffing and puffing breathing" is seen as being mostly unnecessary and tiring.

In 1947 the Maternity Center Association, which had long provided home midwifery service to the poor women of New York (with a safety record better than that of many hospitals) offered a three-year grant to the Yale University Medical School to study the Read method of natural childbirth. The wives of Yale students were educated for natural childbirth. In addition, they were allowed to keep their babies with them in a "rooming-in" program and were encouraged to breast-feed them, an incredible departure from accepted practice of the time.

Yale patients and physicians spread the happy news about the Read method as they moved to other parts of the country. They held public meetings to inform expectant parents. Childbirth education associations were formed, the first three in Milwaukee, Washington, D.C., and Boston. To this day many of the early leaders remain active in the field of childbirth education. Dr. Robert Bradley of Denver, Colorado, made the pioneering statement that husbands, not obstetricians, should be thanked after a joyous birth. He also believed that husbands should be in the delivery room at a natural birth. His colleagues at the time could barely comprehend his statement that 9,000 babies in his practice had been delivered without anesthesia or other drugs.

## The Lamaze Method

Shortly after Dick-Read's work, but entirely independently, the French obstetrician Fernand Lamaze attended an obstetrical conference in Russia where he observed physiologic pain-relief methods and the use of the Pavlovian conditioned-response mechanism. He adapted the technique for his own practice in France, where the drugs used in the United States were considered too dangerous and too expensive and were therefore not generally available. Leon Chertok, a French psychoanalyst, documented in a well-controlled study the shorter labors and the effective pain-relief techniques of Lamaze childbirth. An American woman in France, Marjorie Karmel, brought the Lamaze method to the United States in 1959, and with Elisabeth Bing formed ASPO (the American Society of Psychoprophylaxis in Obstetrics). Over the years, modifications have been made in Lamaze teaching, but the fundamentals remain the same.

During the same year (1960), the International Childbirth Education Association (ICEA) was formed with the goal of improving the childbirth experience, but advocating no one method. The national office is now in Minneapolis with local affiliates across the country. ASPO, with the main office in Washington, D.C., has chapters in many parts of the U.S. Addresses of these two organizations are at the end of the book.

Like the Read approach, the Lamaze method provides education about birth processes, including the importance of relaxing uninvolved muscles. Emotional support is stressed, and husbands learn how to coach their wives in labor.

An active, directive psychological analgesia prevents pain as well as modifying the perception of pain. Read taught the fear-tension-pain connection. Lamaze describes the same phenomenon in different words, explaining that the perception of pain gives the signal for fear and flight, an escape response causing generalized muscular tension. Therefore, Lamaze training conditions the woman to respond to pain with muscular relaxation instead. Also, since stimulation of the cortex of the brain is thought to inhibit pain perception (in the way that a physical ailment is less noticeable during some other engrossing event), controlled breathing during labor is meant to provide a focus of attention away from the pain of labor.

During the weeks before the birth, the husband learns the breathing and relaxation responses to labor contractions, by giving his wife "practice contractions"—for example, putting pressure on a leg muscle to simulate the pressure of the labor contraction. Other preparation methods also use these simulated contractions as rehearsals for labor.

The extra oxygen provided by these special breathing techniques is also thought to prevent pain caused by lack of oxygen to the uterus, which is working hard throughout labor. This method, often called psychoprophylaxis (literally, "mind prevention") has been promoted by childbirth education authorities Majorie Karmel, Elisabeth Bing, Pierre Vellay, M.D., and Irwin Chabon, M.D.

## The Kitzinger Method

Sheila Kitzinger describes her method as a psychosexual approach based on both the Read and Lamaze methods, but it is really closer to the Read teaching with its emphasis on body awareness and response to body signals.

Relaxation is an important part of the Kitzinger method. She describes how anxiety affects involuntary body processes such as heart and digestion as well as labor, and she teaches touch relaxation of arms, head, shoulders, abdomen, legs, wherein the partner touches the woman, while she "relaxes toward" her partner's hands placed on her forehead, legs, shoulders. A slow massage may also be used, and the Stanislavsky techniques of mental imagery—as, for example, a sunny beach, or other scene of her choice—are used to promote muscle relaxation.

As with the Read method, the purpose of the breathing techniques here is for the woman to get in tune with her body, not to distract attention away from the sensations of labor. Instead of the "cleansing breath" marking the beginning and end of each contraction, Kitzinger calls them the "greeting breath" and the "resting breath." She teaches three breathing levels: full-chest breathing with the partner's hands on the back of the lower rib cage, upper-chest breathing with the partner's hands on the upper back, and butterfly breathing with the partner's fingers on her cheeks to focus concentration in this area. During the first stage of labor, or for difficult contractions, light breathing with the lips pursed for the exhalation may be done in a chosen rhythm accenting every few breaths. During the pushing stage, gentle, "sheep's breathing" (light, quick breathing accented by intermittent pushes) is used. Prolonged hard pushing is avoided.

During labor, women are encouraged to walk, lean against heavy furniture, lie on their side with their knees against the chest, kneel on all fours, or sit in a chair with their back supported. The aim of these exercises is to allow the uterus to tilt forward against the abdomen and away from the spine, which helps maintain the baby's heart rate and which uses gravity to encourage the baby to rotate into the correct face-down position for delivery.

Practice contractions are given by the partner by pressing on the flesh of the inner thigh with slow, gradual increase in pressure, followed by decreasing pressure. Partners then reverse roles in this rehearsal for labor so that husband and wife may better understand the other's.

## The Bradley Method

This method, also based on the Read approach and the work of Dr. Robert Bradley, prepares couples for a truly natural birth. The goal is totally unmedicated childbirth, with the mother taking no drugs for three months prior to conception, or during pregnancy, birth, or the breast-feeding period. Of 2,500 couples trained in this method across the country during 1980, 96 percent had a spontaneous unmedicated birth.

The emphasis here is also on tuning in to one's body, both in the first and second stages. There are no levels of breathing; only deep, abdominal breathing throughout labor. Chest breathing is discouraged as being tiring and unnatural. There is no rapid breathing, but women in labor are instructed never to hold their breath at any time during the first stage.

Relaxation is taught with new techniques practiced at each class session. Exercises include tailor sitting, squatting, and other leg separation exercises, the pelvic rock, and the Kegel exercise for the pelvic floor. No exercises are done while lying on the back.

With this method, delivery may occur in a variety of body positions, with semi-squatting the most commonly chosen. The breath is held at times, but only as long as it feels comfortable. Gentle pushing is encouraged. Pain is discussed, and ways of avoiding it are taught. Breast-feeding and nutrition are important components of this method. Prevention of possible problems is addressed in every way possible. Stress-management techniques are taught.

The Bradley method has one thousand active teachers in forty-two states. About one half of the classes are taught by couples.

## The Leboyer Method

The Leboyer method, synonymous with "gentle birth," was pioneered by the French obstetrician, Frederick Leboyer, who suggested more humane treatment of newborn babies. His film, *Gentle Birth,* and book *Birth Without Violence,* documented the responses of babies who were not slapped, held up by the heels, placed on hard surfaces, or given the other rough handling resulting from the need to revive drugged newborns.

Dr. Leboyer instead advocates placing babies immediately after birth in warm water, similar to the uterine environment from which they have just come. Their limbs, weightless in the water, can move more freely, and soft lighting allows them to see their surroundings. They are massaged. The noise level is low, as opposed to the loud voices and clanging metal of the delivery room. The umbilical cord is not cut until the baby is breathing well and can get oxygen through his or her lungs. Babies are nursed. As a result, the loud, anguished cries common to newborns are largely replaced by vocalization, eye contact, body relaxation, and even smiles.

## HOME-BIRTH CLASSES

Home-birth classes do include breathing and comfort techniques, but many tend to deemphasize the importance of breathing exercises, since pain has not been a significant issue in most home births. If there is marked pain in a home birth, it is seen as an indication of a problem possibly requiring hospitalization, not something to be gotten rid of for its own sake. Couples who select a home birth usually fear pain less than they do the routine hospital interventions that could increase the stress on, and the risk to, both parents and baby. Despite this distrust of routine intervention, there is a recognition in home-birth classes that in the case of serious complications some of the hospital procedures can also be life-saving.

Home-birth classes, therefore, are largely devoted to information about normal birth, what could go wrong, how to recognize it, and how to use the hospital if needed. Reasons not to have a home birth are discussed, as are planning the home birth with appropriate people in attendance, how to arrange the home, and what items to have on hand.

Relaxation is considered important, but since this is easier to achieve in a familiar setting surrounded by attendants of one's choice, there is less emphasis on relaxation techniques. Comfortable body positions are suggested: in bed, in an armchair, a bean bag chair, or on large sofa cushions laid on a carpeted floor or mat. The assumption is that the mother will move freely about her house as she desires during labor and eat or drink as she wishes.

Home-birth classes encourage regular breathing patterns during labor, but labor rehearsal is infrequent. In a home birth, or in an alternative birthing center staffed by midwives, it is assumed that the couple has a network of supportive people in watchful attendance throughout the entire labor and in the hours immediately following the birth. Leboyer concepts of gentle birth are likewise assumed.

On-the-spot decisions concerning the birth are made by the couple and those around them. They also work together to promote the mother's comfort. The primary concerns are how the labor goes and how to promote the health of mother and baby, while keeping contact with medical services as needed.

Some home-birth couples feel the need for an additional series of sessions on comfort measures rather than depending so completely on the support people present at the birth. They may also wish to rehearse the labor ahead of time.

## HOSPITAL-SPONSORED CHILDBIRTH CLASSES

The hospital classes, which as might be expected are taught in a hospital, were begun several years after the private classes, which are typically taught in homes. Although the techniques taught in hospital classes are often not the established methods we've been discussing, some classes held in hospitals are privately sponsored and supervised by childbirth education associations. The intentions of hospital classes are generally good, although they are sometimes also seen as a marketing device for hospitals since the number of occupied maternity beds has declined in our post-baby-boom era. The national organizations for childbirth education require their instructors to have between one and two years of training in addition to personal experience in prepared birth. On the other hand, while some hospital or physician-sponsored classes have instructors with a similar background, there are usually no standards, no supervision, and little money spent on such classes. Doctors sometimes recruit office nurses to teach the courses, and many hospital instructors feel restricted to promoting services already offered by the obstetricians and hospitals.

Hospital-sponsored classes do have the advantage of reaching many couples who would otherwise not opt for a prepared birth. However, hospital classes are almost uniformly larger than the recommended ten couples per group, which means that there may be lack of individual attention and inadequate time spent on practicing techniques. Typically, each session should consist of an hour discussing the methods and an hour practicing them. The library of books on childbirth is not available at hospital-sponsored classes.

Often, hospital-sponsored classes, with notable exceptions, are taught by a labor and delivery-room nurse untrained in education for childbirth and with the responsibility of explaining what the hospital does, not what it *should* do, and not the pros and cons of any procedure. Therefore, hospital-sponsored classes can tend to encourage patients to accept what is currently done, making no pretense of addressing controversial issues or the sensitive area of patients' rights.

Parent questions are usually handled with the response, "Ask your doctor," or, "It's done for your safety." Many hospital-sponsored instructors don't tell patients that they have the right to refuse a medication or procedure such as a pubic shave or an enema. Some don't know. In either case, couples are told, "It's up to your doctor."

The nursing branch of the American College of Obstetrics and Gynecology is now moving toward certifying its own instructors. However, this will not solve most of the above problems since hospital instructors, whether certified or not, cannot easily advocate for parents.

## CHILDBIRTH CLASSES: WHAT TO EXPECT

There are some things you can expect in any childbirth class, regardless of the method of preparation taught.

### Instructors

The qualifications of childbirth instructors have often been assumed to include a nursing degree, and many childbirth educators are nurses. However, some are physical therapists, health educators, sociologists, or biologists, and many have no recognized professional background at all. Actually, because childbirth educators are not involved in pathology or medical treatment, a nursing degree may be of little applicability. Rather, what is needed is a thorough knowledge about birth and the techniques used to respond to the forces of birth. The ability to lead group discussions, to enhance parent self-confidence, and to encourage couples to share their feelings with others in the class is vital. A personalized, ombudsman approach can help to counteract the depersonalized, institutional element inevitable in most births.

With rare exceptions, being a parent is a prerequisite for an instructor. If a father can join the teaching team, the class is enriched greatly. Childbirth and parenting involve both parents. Every contraction of labor involves two people, each with a role to play.

The class instructor is most effective when he or she acts as the parents' peer, not an authoritarian expert. Couples are unusually receptive to positive influences during this time, and the classes help to provide accurate information and to encourage confidence that birth, an extraordinary experience, is nevertheless ordinary enough that it does not require medical expertise to accomplish. The instructor may help couples to select medical care according to appropriate criteria, and she may offer labor support in addition, a service that single mothers, especially, may appreciate.

Couples may interview an instructor prior to selecting a class.

## Class Structure

So-called "private" classes are ordinarily held in the informal setting of the instructor's home rather than in a clinical or institutional setting, and are limited to ten couples or fewer.

The class is a two-hour session, often one hour of information and discussion, one hour of floor work for practicing techniques and for rehearsing labor. During this second half, the instructor works with each couple in turn, helping husbands to coach their wives. One or more couples from a previous class may return with their babies to narrate their childbirth experience to the current class of expectant parents.

## Teaching Aids

The instructor usually has a library of childbirth, breast-feeding, and parenting books available for loan. (Recommended reading lists are available from ICEA and other childbirth education associations, as well as the Birth and Life bookstore in Seattle, Washington.) Other teaching aids include:

*The Birth Atlas,* a series of detailed, life-sized photographs of pregnancy, labor, and delivery, is available from the Maternity Center Association in New York City; a model pelvis with a doll (complete with cord and placenta) which can be used to demonstrate the position and descent of the baby is available through childbirth education organizations; a knitted uterus with a drawstring neck to show the dilation of the cervix and the muscular activity of the uterus; and a plastic model from Ross Laboratories in Columbus, Ohio, showing the changing diameter of the cervix as it effaces (flattens) and dilates (opens).

A library of childbirth and breast-feeding films is available from childbirth education associations and affiliated organizations.

## Physician Referral to Classes

Too often, couples wait for the obstetrician to introduce the topic of childbirth classes. Many times, if a doctor does refer a couple, it will be to a hospital-based class. Their medical training still orients physicians to view pregnancy and birth as an "illness" to be treated, not as a natural biological event requiring skills to be learned by those giving birth. To some extent, the obstetrician can see classes as a threat to his or her role as the dispenser of information and treatment, as well as the sacrifice of the benefits of modern obstetrics for some vague idealistic principle. Sometimes childbirth education is seen as a "frill." Although midwives are more likely to refer couples to classes, they too may assume that *they* will tell the parents everything they need to know. However, the general feeling of most physicians and midwives is that couples benefit from childbirth education, and most maintain a list of private or hospital-sponsored classes for couples who ask.

# WHAT IS TAUGHT IN CHILDBIRTH CLASSES

The following pages explain the techniques of relaxation exercises and breathing methods that are generally taught, with some variations, in all childbirth-preparation classes.

The purposes of childbirth education include:

a) To provide information about birth, including the stages of labor and the nature of contractions (as described in the preceding chapter).

b) To teach physical-conditioning exercises.

c) To teach relaxation techniques, including neuromuscular control exercises.

d) To teach methods of breathing to reduce anxiety, provide a focus of attention, promote muscle relaxation, and relieve pain.

e) To demonstrate comfortable body positions to use during labor and delivery.

f) To offer information on general comfort measures.

g) To provide opportunity for labor rehearsals for both partners.

h) To inform expectant parents of their rights and options regarding hospital procedures; to explain the politics of how hospital decisions are made; to help parents communicate effectively with medical-care providers.

i) To give practical information to enhance and facilitate the breast-feeding experience.

j) To make available books and articles to supplement the ten to sixteen hours of class time.

The recurring theme throughout childbirth preparation is that there is no one standard birth or "success" or "failure."

## RELAXATION TECHNIQUES

The stronger the labor contraction, the limper the prepared woman tries to become. However, this total rag-doll limpness is not automatic. It must be learned and practiced.

Nearly forty years ago Edmund Jacobsen, a physiologist, was the first to describe muscular relaxation as a mechanical way of relieving pain. Progressive relaxation involves releasing voluntary muscle groups one at a time, "letting go" of muscles first in the forehead, then in the cheeks, eyes, jaws, neck, chest, shoulders, upper arms, lower arms, wrists, fingers, abdomen, hips, thighs, calves, ankles, and finally toes.

Relaxation can be learned by first tensing a muscle, which increases the awareness of the tension, then letting it go to the maximum extent possible. A deep breath may be taken as a muscle is tensed, then a strong, steady exhalation accompanies the release of the muscle. Focusing on a pleasant mental image, or perhaps visualizing the opening cervix may help relaxation. Or the woman may prefer to focus her eyes on her spouse's face, a photograph, or even a crack in the wall. This fixed focus, combined with the above breathing pattern, promotes relief of muscle tension and feelings of anxiety.

The husband or friend checks the woman's degree of relaxation by gently lifting her hand, rotating her ankle, pressing gently on her thigh, rotating her thigh outward, or checking her calf, shoulder, or arm muscles. This physical contact also serves to provide the woman with non-verbal assurance, and actually promotes muscle relaxation. The woman also needs verbal reassurance that she is relaxing well.

The neuromuscular control exercises teach the woman how to tighten one part of her body while releasing muscles in the rest of the body. The upper part of the body is tightened, while the lower half is released. The left arm and left leg are tightened, the right side of the body is relaxed. The same process is done with the opposite side. Then the left arm and right leg are tightened, the opposing limbs released. Finally, the right arm and opposite leg are then tightened with the opposite limbs relaxed.

These neuromuscular control exercises are done before, not during, labor, since during labor, as the uterus rises up in the abdomen during each contraction, the uterus is the contracting muscle around which all voluntary muscles, especially the abdomen and the vaginal sphincter muscles, are released. The pelvic floor, or Kegel, exercises (described below) help to tone these vaginal muscles, as well as aiding general relaxation.

Why must all muscles be released when only certain muscles are involved in birth? Because tension in one muscle tends to spread to others. Also, any tension tends to disturb the woman's feelings of being in control. The relaxation of uninvolved muscles also helps to save the mother's energy and prevent fatigue.

Arms, legs, back, and hands should be flexed slightly during contractions. Straight limbs are not relaxed.

It's also a good idea for the partner to practice the relaxation exercises while the pregnant woman coaches. This reversal helps each to understand the other's role and is therefore beneficial to both.

## PHYSICAL-CONDITIONING EXERCISES

Physical-conditioning exercises stretch, strengthen, and limber. Designed to increase comfort during both pregnancy and childbirth, they fall into one of four groups: 1) stretching and strengthening inner thigh muscles and limbering pelvic joints; 2) strengthening back and abdominal muscles to relieve backache and to help in carrying the baby in the correct position in the pelvis; 3) increasing control over and strengthening pelvic floor muscles; and 4) promoting comfort during pregnancy. Both partners do the exercises to gain understanding and body awareness of which muscles are being used, which are tense, and which are relaxed.

Swimming and bicycling are among the sports that may be continued throughout pregnancy depending on your level of fitness and whether you have done the activity consistently before pregnancy. Discomfort, fatigue, or pain in the muscles or ligaments indicates the need for rest. Physical contact sports with risk of falling or jarring are generally avoided. Some women do continue to jog well into the pregnancy.

a) *Tailor Sitting*. Sit cross-legged on a firm surface, your back slightly rounded to avoid back strain. If you place your soles together and draw them toward the body, you will get more stretch. The pelvic floor, the muscular tissue between vagina and rectum, can be relaxed and even bulged as you get the feeling of allowing space for the baby to pass through. Some women like to rock from side to side in this position.

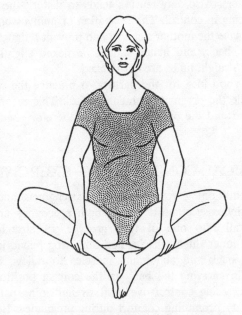

*Tailor sitting*

**b)** *Squatting.* Some women find this difficult to do, and if you have trouble with it, it is not essential. However, since it does serve to open the pelvis to its largest diameter, the exercise can feel good during labor and can be useful in bringing the baby down during delivery. The exercise is used especially in Read-based preparation.

Place your feet about eighteen inches apart with the toes pointed slightly outward. Bend your knees and drop your body downward while keeping your feet flat on the floor. The exercise becomes easier with practice, and you may hang onto your partner's hand or a door knob for balance.

**c)** The *pelvic rock* helps to support the baby in the pelvis during pregnancy, and to strengthen the abdominal and back muscles before and after birth. This exercise, like *tailor sitting* and *squatting,* may also be used during labor for increasing comfort. For "back labor," when contractions are felt mostly in the back, it is usually done in the all-fours position.

To practice the *pelvic rock* lie on your back, press the small of the back against the floor, letting the buttocks lift slowly into the air. Hold the flattened back against the floor with buttocks tightened for several seconds while continuing to breathe. This exercise is easier to do if the knees are raised. After the birth, this exercise helps in bringing back muscle tone and preventing back strain from leaning over the crib.

For the *standing* position, place one hand on your lower back and the other hand over the baby. First tighten the abdominal muscles and tuck the buttocks in with your knees relaxed and your shoulders level. Then release the abdominal and buttock muscles, rocking the pelvis backward. The small of the back should be flattened against the wall as far as possible. (When not doing this exercise, by the way, your buttocks should be tucked under and your abdominal muscles drawn in so that the baby does not rest on a sagging abdomen.)

For the *all-fours* position, get down on your hands and knees and assume a square position with your hands parallel, your shoulders over your hands, and your hips over your knees. As you pull your buttocks under, arch your back like a cat. As you release the buttocks, allow your back to sag (but not really "cave in") as you rock the pelvis. This exercise helps to prevent or relieve back pain in pregnancy and labor.

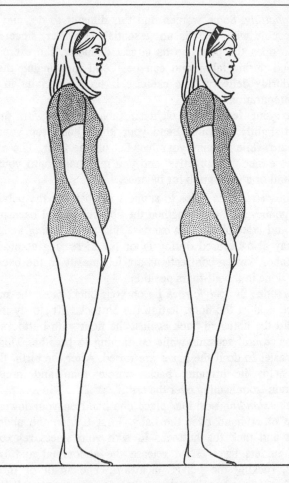

*Pelvic rock in the standing position*

The *stiff-legged walk* tilts the pelvis sideways to exercise the waist muscles. It is also used after delivery to improve muscle tone.

**d)** The *Kegel exercise* was developed forty years ago by Dr. Arnold Kegel for female urinary incontinence as an alternative to surgery, and later recognized as important in female sexual response. Regular practice of this exercise during pregnancy may

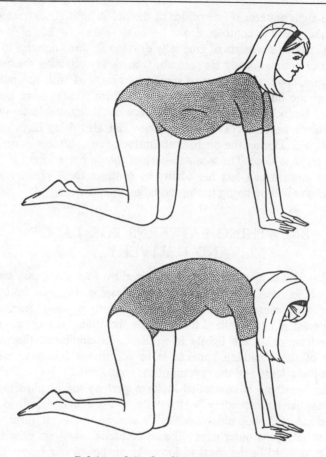

*Pelvic rock in the all-fours position*

help prevent hemorrhoids by improving circulation in that part of the body. More importantly, it promotes elasticity and the ability to release the deep pelvic-floor muscles during birth, thereby decreasing the amount of resistance offered to the baby's head, and easing delivery for mother and baby.

The pelvic floor is the area between the thighs and between the vagina and the rectum. Some of the muscle fibers in this area pass around the rectum and also around the vagina and urethra in a figure-eight pattern. If one orifice of the pelvic floor is contracted, the others tend to contract also.

The exercise consists of gradually drawing in these muscles to a count of approximately six seconds, then slowly releasing them to the same count. The exercise should be practiced with the muscles of the buttocks tightened and with them loosened, as contracted buttocks during the pushing stage can delay the descent of the baby's head. Tight vaginal muscles can also delay birth and cause pain. During the birth, both buttock and sphincter muscles must be kept loose. The woman's partner should remind her.

The woman can test her ability to contract these pelvic-floor muscles at will by trying to stop urination in midstream.

## BREATHING PATTERNS FOR LABOR AND DELIVERY

Your breathing pattern can be affected by your emotional state and can in itself affect your emotions. Gasping, irregular breathing can be caused by panic, and can in turn promote fear. As yoga masters have realized for centuries, breathing, emotions, and body functioning are tightly interrelated. In childbirth, the purpose of the breathing patterns is to coordinate breathing with muscular release and the rhythm of the contraction.

Our breathing is controlled in large part by the diaphragm, a fibrous barrier extending horizontally across the body, dividing the chest and abdominal cavities. When we inhale, it turns up somewhat at the outer edges like an umbrella, when we exhale it moves upward in the chest to force the air out of our lungs. The more deeply we breathe, the farther down into the abdominal cavity the diaphragm extends.

Hyperventilation can occur if breathing is so rapid that it blows off too much carbon dioxide and the body's oxygen-carbon-dioxide balance is altered, thereby affecting the body's acid-base balance and increasing the alkalinity of the mother's blood. The symptoms are dizziness and a tingling in the hands or feet. The remedy is to slow the breathing and even to rebreathe air by cupping your hands over your nose and mouth. With better understanding of childbirth breathing, hyperventilation is seldom a problem. "Huffing and puffing" breathing is little used now. It is not pleasant to do, it dries out the mouth, and can be tiring. Emphasis is rather on relaxation, body position, and emotional support.

Several levels of labor breathing are taught, with small variations depending on the individual class. The general guideline is that breathing should be as relaxed and slow as can be done comfortably, since, as labor progresses, the uterus becomes more sensitive to pressure from the diaphragm and the abdominal muscles.

a) *First-level,* or so-called *abdominal* breathing expands the abdomen like a beach ball with each inhalation and is taught most often in Read-based classes. Some people always do this breathing, but for others normal deep breathing expands only the chest. The so-called abdominal breath is gentle, slow, deep, and comfortable at the rate of five to seven breaths for each contraction. The breath is never held; air exchange is constant. This type of breathing is begun when something more than simple relaxation is required in response to a contraction. It is most often done with breath taken in through the nose and exhaled through pursed lips. For women in hospitals that don't allow water or ice chips during labor, this is the least-drying type of breathing. The abdomen is relaxed, and a hand placed on the rising and falling abdomen helps to center the breathing at this level. Some people use this level for the entire labor. It is the only breathing used in the Bradley method.

Throughout labor, from the beginning of controlled breathing to the very last contraction that brings the baby, each contraction is started with a deep "cleansing" breath and ended with the same deep, complete breath, which sometimes includes a yawn or a relaxing sigh. The purpose is to mark the beginning and end of the contraction and to promote muscle relaxation and a feeling of well-being.

b) *Second-level,* or *chest* breathing may be begun when the contractions become too strong for level one, although some women use level-one breathing for much of the labor. In second-level breathing, the activity is entirely above the waist. The ribs expand and the chest rises to a count of approximately four seconds. The partner can check the rib expansion by placing his

**FIRST-STAGE BREATHING**

**SLOW, DEEP BREATHING**

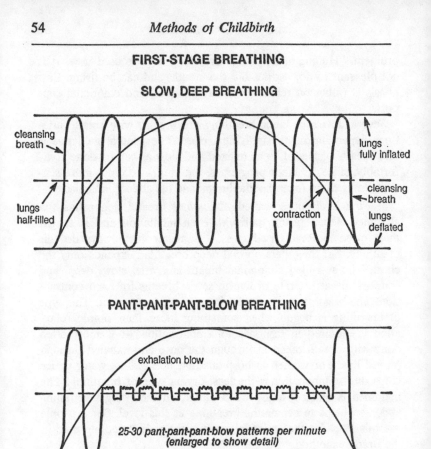

cleansing breath

lungs half-filled

contraction

lungs fully inflated

cleansing breath

lungs deflated

**PANT-PANT-PANT-BLOW BREATHING**

exhalation blow

*25-30 pant-pant-pant-blow patterns per minute (enlarged to show detail)*

**ONE-PANT-ONE-BLOW BREATHING**

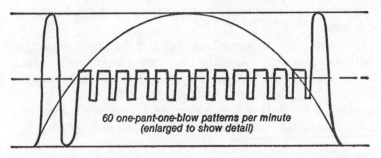

*60 one-pant-one-blow patterns per minute (enlarged to show detail)*

hands on the woman's back. A hand on the rising chest also helps to control chest-level breathing. By putting her hand on her chest she can better feel whether she is indeed doing chest breathing.

c) *Third-level* breathing may be done in a variety of ways, depending largely on individual preference. At times during active labor a woman may do a series of shallow blows through pursed lips, especially if the urge to push begins before dilation is complete.

The newer thinking is less severe than the old, which actively discouraged pushing until the cervix was five fingers dilated, regardless of the urge, to ensure that the cervix was not inflamed or injured by premature pushing. Also, sometimes the obstetrician had not yet been called or was not ready. The newer thinking is that, although premature pushing is undesirable, if the urge is strong and there is only a "lip" of cervix remaining, it is probably desirable to "go with" the urge if pushing does not produce pain, rather than laying guilt on the woman for not waiting for permission. Conversely, if she is fully dilated and feels no urge to push, or if it hurts to push, the woman should do third-level breathing to "blow the contraction away" until she feels the urge.

Active contractions require a rapid, shallow breathing above the level of the sternum or breast bone, almost up into the throat, with pauses between the series of breaths. The rhythm may be a shallow "pant-pant-pant-blow" or, if necessary, a "pant-one, blow-one, pant-one, blow" routine with the head turning from side to side in rhythm with the breathing. (This is the one exception to the rule of keeping a *focal point*.) The rhythm is helpful in providing a focus of concentration and in maintaining general body relaxation. She turns the corners of her lips slightly upward in a smile as she blows shallowly through pursed lips. Turning up the corners of her mouth may seem trivial, but it does help.

Late first-stage breathing is usually very shallow, the chest hardly moving at all. Sometimes a rapid, shallow "humming bird" breathing is done.

d) *Second-stage,* or *expulsion-stage* breathing helps to move the baby down the birth canal. Sometimes the breath is held, sometimes not. Gentle pushing with relaxed buttocks and vagina as taught by the Kegel exercise, instead of a hard, straining push

## SECOND-STAGE BREATHING

### GENTLE PUSHING WITH BREATH HELD INTERMITTENTLY

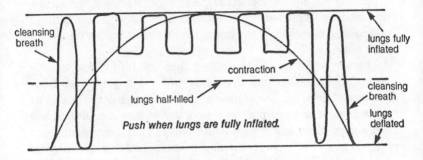

cleansing breath

lungs fully inflated

contraction

cleansing breath

lungs half-filled

lungs deflated

*Push when lungs are fully inflated.*

### GENTLE PUSHING ON EXHALATION BLOW

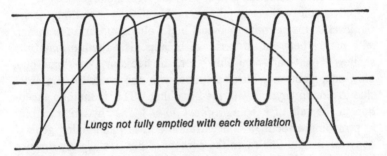

*Lungs not fully emptied with each exhalation*

is now the rule. Speed of delivery is not normally the goal. Some women push only at the peak or as the contraction is subsiding. Most women, if they know the techniques, do not find this stage particularly uncomfortable. In fact, they generally find it the best part of the labor and often really enjoy it.

For the last contraction, a pushing breath is not used, to avoid possible tearing of the vaginal tissues at delivery. A shallow pant or blow allows the uterus alone to produce enough pressure without aid from the diaphragm.

## COMFORT DURING LABOR

### Body Positions

*Comfortable body positions* for labor and birth include almost any position other than the supine, or flat-on-the-back position, which can cause painful overstretching of the abdominal muscles, as well as back strain, both of which may cause pain and therefore tightening of the vaginal muscles. Most serious, the pressure of the baby on a major blood vessel in this position interferes with the blood supply to the uterus, reducing the amount of oxygen that reaches the baby and causing the woman's heart to beat faster. Despite the wealth of research on this topic, one can still see supine women in hospital labor and delivery rooms, lying flat on their backs while pushing out their babies against the force of gravity.

Comfortable body positions during labor include *tailor sitting*

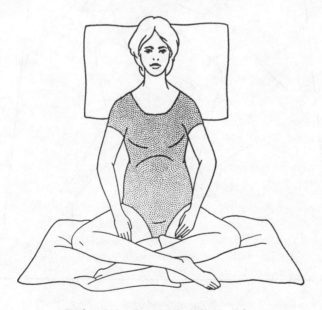

*Tailor sitting for comfort during labor*

with a pillow under each knee and the back supported, *side positions* with a pillow between the knees to prevent hip pain, and *semi-sitting* positions with a pillow under each knee and pillows under the head and shoulders. Comfort is further increased in this last position if a pillow is placed under each elbow, and relaxation is aided if all the joints are slightly flexed, and the hands are curved into a relaxed position. The woman's partner should check frequently during contractions for relaxed hands, arms, and legs.

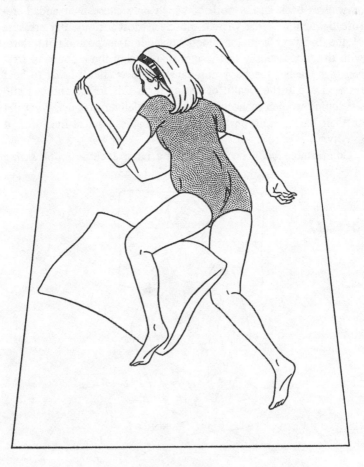

*The side position*

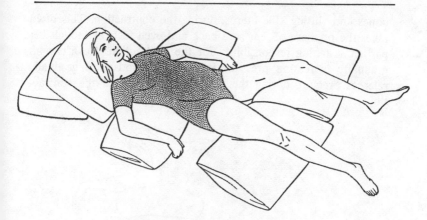

*A variation of the semi-sitting position*

In a variation of the semi-sitting position, two pillows are placed behind the head and shoulders, with a pillow also under each knee. Here the knees are somewhat apart and rotated outward.

At times during labor or birth the woman may get into a *squatting* position with her heels down to ease pressure on her back or hips or get up onto *all fours* for a while to promote a relaxed abdomen and general comfort. Labor is helped both in degree of comfort and progress of cervical dilation or descent by *standing* and *walking* occasionally. Changes of position promote comfort and increase circulation, and moving around the room or walking often helps the woman to feel more like a person giving birth instead of like a hospital patient. However, the use of electronic fetal monitors (described in Chapter Four) prevents the woman from getting out of bed, and may even inhibit her mobility in bed. Leaning forward against her partner's shoulders may also promote comfort, as will a trip to the bathroom to empty her bladder. She may want to walk to the sink and sponge her face or look out the window. Sitting in a rocking chair is often comfortable. Gentle massage of the abdomen, known as *effleurage* in Lamaze training, may feel good to some women. Firm but *gentle pressure* against one or both sides of the uterus, not the abdomen, helps to support the uterus and relax the abdominal muscles. "Abdominal lifting" involves supporting both sides of the abdomen just above the hip bones and "lifting" the uterus, during the contraction. This often takes the pressure off her sore back and even feels as though her partner is taking responsibility for the contraction. He lifts with gradually increasing pressure for thirty seconds and gradually releases pressure during the next thirty seconds of the contraction.

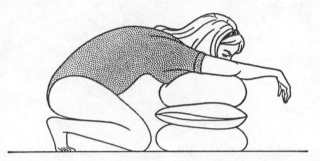

*The kneeling position*

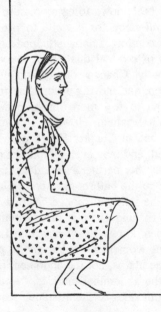

*Squatting*

*Three ways of relieving backache during labor*

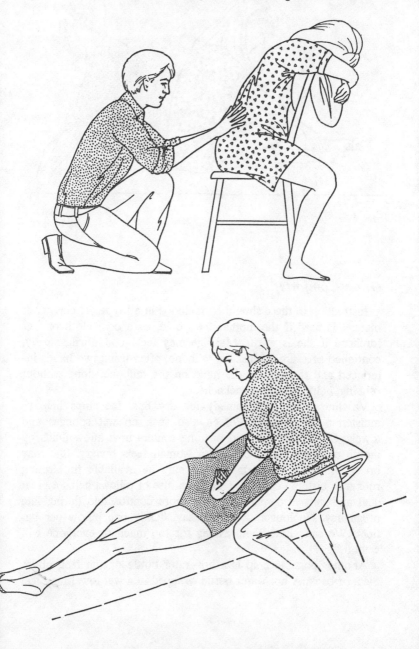

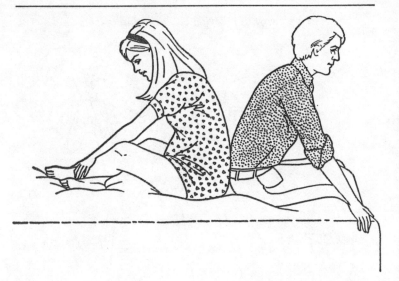

## Other Comforts

Instruction in these should be included in all types of classes. A blanket is used if the mother feels cold, or a cool cloth on her forehead if she is warm. Massage may feel good. Firm, steady, continued pressure against the tailbone, often using two hands interlaced and the heel of the hand on the tailbone, done without rubbing, helps to relieve backache.

Vaseline is the best remedy for dry lips. Ice chips help to moisten a dry mouth. Women also suck on wet sponges and towels. Many hospitals and birthing centers now allow fluids by mouth or even a light meal if a woman feels hungry. She may brush her teeth. A warm shower may be available in birthing rooms or birthing centers. The liberal use of pillows helps a great deal and may also make sleeping more comfortable during late pregnancy. No longer do nurses say, "Only one pillow per patient. We can't have them asking for too much or everyone will want it."

Another possible help is a hot-water bottle on the feet, abdomen, or back. A hot-water bottle wrapped in a wet towel may feel good, and placed against the vagina during the second stage may help to relax the pelvic floor for delivery.

Hospitals do not have hot-water bottles; therefore these must be brought from home along with a robe and warm socks for air-conditioned facilities, and ready-to-eat food for the father during labor—perhaps also for the mother, depending on circumstances.

*Clothes* are usually exchanged for a hospital johnny and a plastic bracelet with an identifying number. If a hospital gown is worn, the woman should ask for two of them, wearing one with the opening in front and the other with the opening in back so she can feel free to move around the labor unit without exposing herself. Or she may bring her own robe, or even stay in her own clothes. Many people assume that the gown is for the purpose of sterility, but this is not so. Shoes, socks, and slippers are useful, although hospital slippers may be available.

One of the most important comfort measures of all is to *keep the bladder empty*. Since bladder capacity is greatly reduced by the size of the uterus, the woman must get up to go to the bathroom at least every two hours, especially if there is an intravenous drip. But even if there is no IV or anything given by mouth, the bladder must be emptied, as a full bladder can delay the progress of labor by preventing the descent of the baby's head. Also, bladder pressure, which ranges from a dull ache to a sharp pain, is frequently misinterpreted as labor pain that won't go away between contractions. If walking to the bathroom is impossible because of electronic monitoring equipment, a bedpan can be used.

Finally, a serene, non-intrusive environment is essential to the mother's comfort throughout labor.

# Chapter Three

---

# MEDICATION AND ANESTHESIA FOR CHILDBIRTH

Pain-killers used in childbirth are a mystery to many people. If an unprepared couple should request that the mother be "knocked out," there is often the mistaken assumption that she will be anesthetized for the whole labor and delivery. This is not the case. However, there are drugs given to relieve pain in labor, and there are several types of anesthesia used for delivery.

It was early noted that narcotics, barbiturates, and inhalation anesthesia could produce a stuporous baby slow to turn from blue to pink as the lungs inflate for the first time. In fact, this condition was observed so routinely that it came to be viewed as normal newborn behavior. However, more recent work has shown that this is not normal, and that the effects can last beyond the delivery room into early hours, days, and weeks of life, and may even be permanent. The American Foundation for Maternal and Child Health reports that one out of every ten American children is learning-disabled, and that one out of every thirty-five children is eventually diagnosed as mentally retarded. It is now widely believed that drugs given during labor and delivery, by interfering with the oxygenation of the child's brain cells, can cause learning disability. The recognition of these possible problems, along with the desire of parents to be active participants in birth, has resulted in a decrease in the use of drugs as well as in lower dosages.

The Committee on Drugs of the American Academy of Pediatrics states that no drug administered to childbearing women has been proven safe for the unborn child.

The Food and Drug Administration does not guarantee the safety of any drug it approves as safe. In fact, the FDA does not even have a specific definition of safety. A pharmaceutical manufacturer filing a new drug application is not required to establish its long-term effects on the subsequent neurologic, mental, or physical development of the child in order to gain approval for use in childbirth. Yet physicians depend on the FDA to inform them of the safety of the drugs they prescribe.

Moreover, the American College of Obstetrics and Gynecology (ACOG) establishing a Washington, D.C., office in addition to its Chicago headquarters, works to influence governmental agencies, including the FDA, in ways that are sometimes opposed to the goals of various consumer groups. For example, ACOG has opposed making package inserts from drug manufacturers available to patients, arguing that patients: 1) will not understand the information, and 2) will, as a result of the inserts, worry about their medications instead of trusting their doctors.

Taking a look backward at the origins of medicated "knock 'em out, drag 'em out" childbirth, we must remember that the major reason that middle- and upper-class women first came to hospitals to have their babies was to get the "twilight sleep" available only in hospitals and advertised in ladies' magazines. The feminism of the twenties encouraged women to escape from domesticity and to hail these changes, which distanced them from biology and parenting. No longer were women satisfied by drinking cordials to take the edge off labor pain. They wanted to be unconscious. Most remembered nothing for many hours before and after birth. At first, most doctors were reluctant to use anesthesia for birth, but women demanded it, and physicians soon discovered that there were advantages for them as well: Their presence during labor was no longer required, and patients seldom complained about any aspect of their birth experiences.

Gradually, physicians began to feel that their role was to manage labor from afar rather than to aid women in labor, and to "deliver" the baby rather than to assist at the birth. Drugs were given on admission. Some women reported never feeling a single labor contraction.

Twilight sleep was also a way of coping with fear of birth. Women were afraid of the birth process as well as the accompanying pain. Safe Cesareans were only beginning to be available in the 1920s, and there were no antibiotics until the 1940s. Blood transfusions were still new. Venereal disease was prevalent. Crowded, unsanitary living conditions of the industrial revolution were not conducive to health. Upper-class women exercised little and were often laced into tight corsets that deformed their rib cages and tended to compress the abdominal organs. Births were frequent and contraception virtually unavailable. Nutrition was often poor for all classes, and infant deaths from communicable diseases were numerous. Women could easily welcome oblivion at birth as somehow safer in addition to less painful.

Women of that era had another reason to fear the pain of childbirth. When midwives were largely replaced by European-trained physicians during the 1800s, the doctors brought to this country a tool that the midwives did not have—forceps. Although forceps could deliver babies faster, they were often painful—and used without anesthesia. And though sometimes forceps were needed to deliver babies who could not be expelled unaided, sometimes even high forceps were used, both in the home and the hospital, when the baby's head had barely entered the birth canal. As a result, the women needed pain relief more than ever.

In 1920 Dr. Joseph DeLee of Chicago introduced the prophylactic, or preventive, forceps procedure and the prophylactic episiotomy to enlarge the birth opening. The forceps were described as preventing danger to the infant's brain. The episiotomy's purpose was to allow the introduction of the forceps.

DeLee's theory and practice formed the foundation for modern obstetrical practice until only recently. The woman was sedated and her cervix allowed to dilate, while the fetal heart was monitored by stethoscope. Ether was given when the fetus entered the birth canal. It was stipulated that the second, or pushing, stage should last no more than two hours. A cut of several inches was then made through the skin and muscle of the perineum (the area between the vagina and anus) and forceps were used. Ergot or a derivative was then used to contract the uterus. The placenta (afterbirth) was extracted by hand, and the woman was stitched. Hospitals soon made this procedure commonplace.

Actually, this method of handling birth is still common today, except that an anesthesia other than ether is used, and Pitocin, rather than ergot, is used to contract the uterus. This routine is sometimes called the "cut, pull, sew" method.

The anthropologist Margaret Mead, who had observed birth in other cultures, strove mightily in the 1940s to obtain natural childbirth and a family-centered delivery for her only child. The most she could negotiate was an unanesthetized birth. After delivery, her baby was immediately transported to the central nursery like all the rest.

In the following chapters it will become more evident that "everything is connected to everything else." For instance, anesthesia may require forceps. Forceps may require an episiotomy. Anesthesia also prohibits the mother from holding her baby after birth.

In general, anesthesia contributed heavily to the dehumanization of maternity care. The resultant roles of passive female and absent husband placed all decisions about birth in the hands of medical experts. The physician-patient relationship was, and still tends to be, based on a father-daughter pattern, where she may be expected to trust him and defer to him. In reality, the couple is hiring the obstetrician to perform a service, and the relationship might better be one of consultant to client or, perhaps, of friend to friend. Although untrained men (i.e., husbands) were at first seen as weak and useless at birth, trained men (i.e., doctors) were seen by many as being more competent than women, whether those women were midwives, obstetricians, or nurses, and certainly more competent than the anesthetized woman recumbent on the table.

Later, spinal anesthesia was introduced, allowing women to be awake during birth. Often, however, the labor drugs were given in such dosages that the woman was already unconscious before the spinal was given. Also, women sometimes refused to look even when offered the opportunity to view the birth through a mirror in the delivery room. The sight of birth was, if not frightening, at least indelicate. Birth still belonged to the professionals.

The use of drugs and anesthesia has affected almost every aspect of obstetrical care. Many of the rituals associated with anesthetized birth have continued even after women were no longer routinely rendered unconscious and/or partially paralyzed during the birth of their children. For example, family members were originally not present because the patients were drugged. Women were alone in labor rooms, often several to a room, except for an occasional check by a nurse of the vital signs, which included maternal pulse, respiration, and fetal heart rate. No food or drink was allowed during labor. Communication with drugged laboring women was almost impossible. Ties and bed rails were standard for labor, and stirrups and stout leather handcuffs were used for every birth. Babies were transported to busy central nurseries and not shown to mothers until twelve or even twenty-four hours after birth. Later, when women were awake and unmedicated, and no longer desiring assembly-line maternity care, an unsubstantiated rationale often developed against parent objections to routines that had been developed for irresponsible drugged mothers and absent fathers.

The rationale went as follows:

a) Anesthetized birth was "safer," even if not needed for pain, because it prevented the "pounding of the baby's head against the perineum," the assumption being that the force of the uterine contractions against unyielding vaginal tissues was potentially dangerous. Better, it was assumed, to immobilize her, relax her uterus and voluntary muscles with anesthesia, and use forceps, so that the force of the traction would be under physician control.

b) There was no need to provide continuing nursing care during labor. The cost would be prohibitive and, besides, if patients felt pain they could be drugged. There was no need to pay for hand-holding. The receiving of prescribed drugs was, for many women, their sole individual contact with the nursing staff except for a periodic fetal heart check. Because nurses could not communicate with drugged women, they frequently found the obstetrical unit a boring place to work. This kind of obstetrical care persists in some hospitals and obstetric practices even though women are awake and are able to communicate and participate in making decisions about their baby's birth.

Awake, unanesthetized women faced the same lack of support as drugged women. There was no need for fathers to be present when women were unconscious. When they were awake, they were told that husbands would bring in germs and might faint. A legal brief filed in California in the 1960s by a lawyer, Fay Stender, documented that of the 40,000 men who had been in labor and delivery rooms with their wives, none had fainted, brought infections, or sued the doctor or hospital.

c) Bed rails were to be used because they gave the patient something to hang onto. Handcuffs would keep her from falling off the table, or from touching the birth area, the baby, or the sterile sheets draped over her legs and abdomen. Some said it gave her a place to put her hands. Stirrups held the legs of the anesthetized woman in a position convenient for the obstetrician.

d) The woman could have nothing by mouth during the hours of labor, even a sip of water, because of the possible use of gas anesthesia.

e) Even if undrugged, it was believed, the woman would be too tired to take immediate interest in the baby. Mother love develops later, it was hypothesized. During her hospital stay she would be too tired to care for her baby and probably wasn't competent if a first-time mother. Also, she was in the hospital for a vacation from womanly chores. Infant care in the hospital was viewed as none of the mother's business.

f) Patient rights continued to be violated even when most women were no longer rendered helpless and husbands were present. Now, however, the problems were more subtle as patients were channeled into the interventionist obstetrical care associated with the newer types of anesthesia, such as epidural anesthesia. Scare tactics were often used by hospital staff who disseminated misinformation that was, in reality, no more substantiated than the oft-ridiculed "old wives' tales."

g) The possibility of a complication from medication or anesthesia was judged acceptable because the level of risk was within the parameters acceptable to the profession. Even after research indicated otherwise, women were told that drugs were "perfectly safe." Accountability was virtually impossible, since sluggish babies with poor color were seen as "normal," and diagnoses of minimal brain damage, seizures, cerebral palsy, learning disability, and hyperactivity often didn't come until years after birth.

Today, prepared childbirth and childbirth classes are accepted and encouraged. Husbands or friends may be present during labor, birth, and afterward. Labor medications are now used minimally or not at all. Communication with the majority of maternity nursing staffs has vastly improved. The use of handcuffs for delivery is rare. Parents have access to their infants and breast-feeding is encouraged.

However, communication with many obstetricians remains difficult. Parents are frequently uninformed about the risks as well as the benefits of obstetrical interventions. Many women are still confined to bed with nothing allowed by mouth throughout their labor. Regional anesthesia is still widely used for normal birth as are stirrups and forceps. Many parents are still denied immediate access to their newborn children.

## PAIN RELIEF

Women who have not had preparation for birth, or incomplete preparation, can expect to receive either epidural anesthesia (described below) begun during active labor, or spinal anesthesia for the last one or two contractions. Sometimes, however, caring and capable obstetricians and nurses will coach an unprepared couple through contractions without drugs or anesthesia.

Anesthetized birth, with the exception of local anesthesia, usually requires that the woman lie flat on her back, even though sitting, standing, or squatting is suggested by both anatomy and the law of gravity, and maintains oxygenation of the baby. Since spontaneous birth is usually impossible under general or spinal anesthesia, the obstetrician must use either forceps or strong pressure on the abdomen. An incision is generally made to enlarge the vagina for delivery.

Ironically, women who have birth experiences of this type may find that their fears about childbirth are increased, because they do not know what happens during birth and have no control over what happens. They come out of anesthesia with very sore bottoms and often have temporary difficulty walking as well as emptying their bladders and rectums. Spray-on analgesics, sitz baths, laxatives, and oftentimes catheters are necessary as a result of this type of birth.

However, pharmacological methods of pain relief can be valuable for use in childbirth. They can relieve parents' anxiety because pain relief is given promptly upon request. No woman need experience more pain than she wishes to accept in her desire to participate as fully as possible in birth. Parents can learn what to expect from various drugs to relieve their fear of the unknown and to use these aids wisely.

There are two major types of pain relief. *Medications* for labor are analgesic drugs, which raise the pain threshold to effect relief. Narcotic substances are most often used for this.

*Anesthesia* is a substance introduced into the body to produce an unconscious state or to cause numbness in a certain part of the body. *General anesthesia,* now rarely used in vaginal birth, produces unconsciousness and may be introduced as inhalation (gas) anesthesia, such as ether or cyclopropane, or by needle into a blood vessel, as is pentothal. Sodium pentothal, however, is considered too dangerous for use in childbirth. *Regional anesthesia,* such as spinal and epidural anesthesia, blocks sensations from a wide area of the body. *Local anesthesia* numbs only the area immediately surrounding the injection, as, for example, in the dental office when Novocain is injected before a tooth is filled.

In general, *analgesic medications* are used during the first (cervical dilation) stage of labor. Most types of *anesthesia* are given during the second (expulsive) stage of labor, when the baby moves down the birth canal just before delivery, since anesthesia inhibits or stops labor contractions.

## MEDICATIONS USED FOR LABOR

Every medication the mother takes passes through the placenta to the baby. Originally given as pills, labor medications are now usually injected into the buttock by a nurse after being prescribed by the physician. The hospital is especially efficient in the distribution of medications, and until the advent of educated, prepared childbirth with its pillows, warm showers, and other comfort techniques, these drugs were the only method available to promote comfort and relieve labor pain. In fact, in the past drugs were routinely used even when women reported feeling no pain at all. Some women were given drugs on admission and do not recall having felt a single contraction.

Dosages are variable. A relaxed woman receiving reassurance usually responds readily to a small dose, while a tense, frightened, uninformed woman with no spouse or friend for support will require more. Because there is no way of "undoing" the effects of a drug once it is given, childbirth class instructors teach couples to start with a minimum dose, then ask for more if needed. All medications can decrease the mother's alertness and sense of being in control, and all can result in feelings of weakness, fatigue, and perhaps dizziness.

The original famed "twilight sleep" was achieved with a combination of morphine and an amnesic drug, but the use of morphine in childbirth was discontinued many years ago. The most common drugs in current or recent use are described below. Note that all have medical uses other than in childbirth.

*Narcotics* are substances that act to raise the pain threshold. The one most commonly used in labor has been Demerol. This is an effective analgesic whose effects are evident within minutes after injection. The side effects are fatigue, drowsiness or weakness, and possible dizziness, which can make concentration on a focal point and breathing techniques difficult. A starting dose as low as 25 milligrams may give adequate pain relief. Normally not enough is given to produce sleep. However, many women with no medication do sleep between, or even during, some contractions, especially if labor occurs during the night. The effects of Demerol last from two to four hours, often longer than is needed. It passes through the placenta to the baby and can produce a sluggish baby of poor color. It acts to depress infant breathing.

Nisentil, a short-acting synthetic narcotic in use for many years, was withdrawn from the market in 1980.

Barbiturates act to produce sleep. Seconal or, less frequently, Nembutol is used. No direct pain relief is provided by barbiturates, but the sedative effect, tending to produce sleep, can provide pain relief indirectly. Seconal may be given to help the woman sleep if she is in early labor and cannot relax in the hospital environment, but under these circumstances she should be in her own home anyway, unless hospital procedures such as breaking the bag of waters have already been done. Barbiturates do depress the baby, even if they are given a day or two before birth, and most women prefer not to have them. A sleepy baby can result with accompanying depressed sucking response, slowed weight gain, and altered brain patterns. Effects last several days until the baby's immature liver can metabolize the barbiturate.

*Tranquilizers* are used to relieve anxiety. Valium, Sperine, or other substances are occasionally given to help a tense woman relax her muscles, an important part of pain relief, and to allay anxiety. They may also be used to potentiate the effect of other drugs. Understanding birth and practicing deep muscle relaxation make less likely the need for tranquilizers. They do pass through the placenta.

*Amnesics* remove memory. Scopolamine, introduced from Germany in 1916, was used regularly for more than fifty years, and is still used occasionally in obstetrical practices and hospitals to "knock out" patients. This type of delivery has largely disappeared because mothers, now less frightened of childbirth, usually wish to be awake and aware for the arrival of their children. Heavily medicated birth, first declared unsafe by proponents of natural childbirth, is now widely considered even by physicians to pose an unacceptable risk to both mother and child.

The use of Scopolamine for most deliveries in this country for fifty years is a dark chapter in obstetrical practice. This drug did not relieve pain, and often actually increased it because of the agitation it frequently caused in the mother. If a woman were in pain, her cries for help might be ignored because the nursing personnel assumed she was only hallucinating under the influence of "scope," a hallucinogen with chemical properties similar to those of LSD.

Occasionally the woman became stuporous instead of thrashing about, especially when Scopolamine was combined with Seconal and Demerol, which it usually was. She felt pain, but couldn't remember it later. If she spoke, her words made no sense and she would have no memory of them when the drug wore off. Occasionally, partial memory remained, and then the woman worried about what she had said while under the influence of the drug.

Scoped women were usually kept in a common labor room, tied to their beds with the side rails up. Sometimes, wondering about their bruises the next day, they assumed that childbirth must be an awful, agonizing process. Scopolamine, however, was rarely discussed with women or described in the ladies' magazines.

Physicians liked the drug because it lightened their workload, and because it allowed them to assure women that they would feel no pain and remember nothing. They did not dare to use enough narcotics and barbiturates to cause total oblivion, even with such orders as 100 milligrams of Demerol, 100 milligrams of Seconal combined with a third drug, a tranquilizer such as Thorazine, the order to be repeated once again with the same or smaller dose after several hours of labor. And this was only for labor. For the birth, women also had anesthesia. Sometimes, if she had not delivered within twenty-four hours of the onset of labor, the opinion was that the woman had overdosed to a degree that labor could not progress, in which case the every-four-hours medications were then halted. Next day the patients regularly thanked their doctors for taking such good care of them, and requested the same treatment for their next baby.

Scopolamine is still used today in small doses for non-obstetric conditions. It can be used as one of the preoperative medications before surgery, where it is valued because it helps dry the patient's mouth so that there will be less saliva produced during unconsciousness. Over-the-counter sleep preparations may also contain small amounts of Scopolamine.

All four types of medications, including Scopolamine, were routinely used for labor until almost 1970. The woman, shortly after being admitted to the hospital, was given a narcotic, a barbiturate, an amnesic, and a tranquilizer. This use of medication, in fact, was a reason for the traditionally rough handling of the newborn. The holding up of the naked baby by the heels in the cool room, the shaking or even spanking was considered necessary to revive the drugged newborn and initiate breathing. Holding babies up by the heels was also thought necessary "to drain the mucus" from the infant's throat and mouth. These practices, too, continued into the 1970s, even after the use of the medications began to decline.

Medications, in the more conservative manner they are used today, do have a place in childbirth. They are used most effectively when an informed couple makes the decision. A small dose of Demerol or perhaps a tranquilizer is the usual preference. A common time to assess the possible need for drugs is at approximately 5 centimeters of cervical dilation, when labor is well established. If at this time the woman feels no stronger uterine sensations than she is willing to accept, it is probable that there will be no need for medication. Transition, the most painful time, is ahead; but it is the shortest stage, seldom over forty-five minutes, even for a first labor. The second, expulsive stage is normally, and with proper pushing technique, the least painful part of the entire labor.

Nurses are those most in contact with patients; however, the patients are not theirs, but the physicians'. Nurses may not ordinarily refuse to carry out a physician's order, although they can be liable for carrying out an erroneous order. Couples may be irritated at the nurse who keeps popping in to offer Demerol, but only the patient can refuse the obstetrician's order. The drug order is usually written "PRN," meaning medication as the patient requests. Husband, friends, or childbirth educators who may be present may make a suggestion or offer information, but the woman herself must be the one to make the decision whether to accept or refuse medication.

If women accept medication after being informed that they have hours yet to go with the worst yet to come, and then give birth an hour later, they can feel cheated and angry. No one can accurately predict the length of labor. However, the decision to take medication during the first stage may make a woman less likely to request otherwise unnecessary anesthesia for the birth.

Seldom do couples feel a sense of "failure" for accepting medication if all physiological help and comfort measures are first used and if the couple themselves make the decision. However, when the birth experience is wrested from their control and they feel compelled to accept unwanted medication, their anger and depression can be long lasting.

## ANESTHESIA USED FOR CHILDBIRTH

Currently, obstetrical patients have more control over the labor medications they receive than they do over the anesthesia they are given. The reasons are several. One is that hospital obstetrical clinics, in which a single fee is paid for total obstetrical care, including doctor and hospital, will be staffed by resident obstetricians and anesthesiologists under supervision. Since these physicians-in-training need experience with medical techniques, there is a greater likelihood that a woman will be given anesthesia unless she expresses an objection. According to one couple who had their baby at a teaching hospital, "Those anesthesiology residents were like a pack of wolves waiting in the wings for us to let them put in an epidural or accept a spinal in the delivery room."

Also, the couple does not meet the anesthesiologist until labor is in progress, and usually they have no choice about who it is. In teaching hospitals, it is most often an anesthesia resident under supervision of a staff anesthesiologist. The anesthesiologist may ask at the beginning of labor what anesthesia the woman wishes. Sometimes, however, the woman is asked at the time of transition, the most difficult although shortest part of labor, and the time when the woman desires encouragement in her efforts but is also most vulnerable to suggestion that someone else take over and do it for her. Or the first contact between patient and anesthesiologist may not even be until the delivery room, where the obstetrician may have already arranged for a spinal.

Birth has, until recently, taken place almost entirely in the delivery room, which is actually an operating room. The obstetrician is in charge of what happens in the delivery room, and physicians haven't been in the habit of asking the patient on the table what she wants. Rather, he has seen it as his role to make decisions, and this has been important to his feeling of professional competence. In obstetrics, the doctor-patient relationship has changed to an extent, but some obstetricians may become angry when their patients see themselves as colleagues in the event of birth instead of as compliant patients. It is therefore crucial for parents to have a good understanding of the uses of anesthesia.

The woman and her mate also have to keep in mind that the second stage of labor and the delivery itself are normally the least painful parts of childbirth, with tissue numbness and rectal pressure the predominant sensations. Obstetricians, as well as women, had difficulty for years in accepting the fact that the actual birth is not the most painful part of the process. Many women have been allowed to remain unmedicated for labor, then given anesthesia at the very end. Women eventually informed their physicians that the end was the "good part," but even then many doctors assumed that the individual woman either had a high pain threshold or was being a martyr.

More directly to the point is the obstetrician's assumption that he is there to "do the delivery." How can he, and obstetricians are still predominantly male, introduce forceps, and many obstetricians still do only forceps deliveries, without anesthesia? And how can he introduce the forceps into an intact, uncut vagina? (The assumption is that the forceps will not fit unless the episiotomy incision is made.)

Gradually many obstetricians learned that episiotomies can be done, in many cases, without anesthesia, because the pressure from the baby's head numbs the surrounding tissues adequately. However, childbirth educators, women's health groups, and informed obstetricians usually suggest the use of Novocain, or more typically Xylocaine, if an episiotomy is to be done. This local anesthesia is sufficient, and the explanation, "We give the spinal for the episiotomy," is now seldom heard.

Many obstetricians still find it difficult to understand why women object to regional anesthesia such as a spinal as long as they can remain awake. Obstetricians may even define a "natural childbirth" as one where the woman is awake, regardless of the medications and regional or local anesthesia given. These obstetricians still do not see how a woman can enjoy the pushing stage and wish to feel, if possible, the descent of the baby under the control of her own expulsive efforts, or why she desires the experience of giving birth instead of "being delivered."

The anesthesia can affect every aspect of the birth, including the woman's ability to sit, to squat, to turn onto her side, to move into the delivery position of her choice—the latter a high priority among many informed couples.

Anesthesia can also affect the woman's ability to push her baby down. It takes from her the decision about the speed and the time of birth. It may affect how the hours after birth are spent. Usually, it indirectly removes from the couple the decision about whether to have an episiotomy. It may even, in the case of the epidural, affect whether or not a Cesarean or "abdominal" birth occurs.

Most obstetricians do not wish to have their role become that of a midwife or birth attendant but rather that of decision-maker and "doer." Anesthesia has justified their presence at many, many births.

## Types of Anesthesia

### LOCAL

There are four types of *local anesthesia*.

The first, "nature's anesthesia," or pressure anesthesia, has already been mentioned. It is usually effective unless the second stage is short or rushed, when there is less time for the vaginal tissues and pelvic floor to become numb. It works best with slow, gentle pushing. If an episiotomy is to be done without Novocain or Xylocaine, the baby's head must be entirely down with most of the top of the head (called the occiput) visible to provide sufficient numbness. A local anesthesia described below must almost always be used for suturing even if done immediately after birth.

Novocain or Xylocaine may be injected near the entrance to the vagina in one or more places. It is placed just under the skin and is ordinarily very effective. It does not affect the woman's control over her body in any way. She can still move, sit, and push her baby out. If she is to have an episiotomy she will ask for this type of anesthesia.

*Pudendal Block* anesthesia is given by injection of a substance such as Xylocaine into the pudendal nerves on both sides of the vagina. The needle goes in more deeply, but causes no distress to the woman. The vagina is numbed, allowing the use of forceps if necessary.

With the pudendal, the woman can still move and walk. She can push her baby down the birth canal. Only the vagina and surrounding tissues are anesthetized.

*Paracervical Block:* Here the anesthetizing substance is injected into the cervix at time intervals of approximately one hour during the first stage of labor. Although the cervix has few pain fibers, the paracervical block does sometimes help a tight cervix to dilate during the first stage. Its use is now minimal because the anesthetizing substance gets into the baby's bloodstream through the placenta and tends to slow the baby's heart rate. (This anesthesia may also be used for the gynecological procedure of dilation and curettage of the uterus, better known as a "D and C." Women who do not wish to be unconscious for the procedure may request a paracervical block.)

### REGIONAL ANESTHESIA

Regional anesthesia affects more of the body than does local anesthesia. There are several types used for childbirth, some of which are also used for surgery.

*Spinal anesthesia* is used for many surgical procedures in which waist-to-toe immobility and loss of sensation are desired. The anesthesia takes effect moments after administration and usually lasts several hours, the length of time depending partly on the amount of anesthesia used. As the spinal wears off, the woman will be able to move her toes first, then her legs, then the rest of the affected area.

Many women who ask for a spinal assume mistakenly that it is given during labor to alleviate painful contractions. In fact, a spinal is *given for the last contraction or next-to-last contraction,* just minutes before birth, usually when the baby's head is visible. It must be given at the end of labor because it inhibits contractions and stops the labor, and even so, forceps or fundal (abdominal) pressure is required to deliver the baby.

Spinals are given by introducing an anesthetizing substance such as Xylocaine into the fluid surrounding the spinal cord. The patient lies on her side curled into the fetal position to maximize the space between the vertebrae. She feels only a prick as the anesthesia is given. (Sometimes more than one attempt must be made.) Then she is quickly rolled onto her back and placed in stirrups, the effects of the anesthesia evident almost immediately. She must be watched constantly by the anesthesiologist who checks her vital signs, and is assured that the muscles of respiration are not affected.

Like all drugs, the spinal anesthesia passes through the placenta, but, because it is given so late, its direct effects on the baby are almost non-existent. Indirect effects are reduced blood circulation and therefore diminished oxygen to the baby because of the sudden drop in blood pressure associated with spinal anesthesia. However, the baby is usually born promptly after the anesthesia is given.

At one time in American obstetrics, especially during the 1950s and sixties, when babies were being delivered on an assembly-line basis, women about to deliver were given a spinal to hold them until the obstetrical staff could attend them. The delay gave the obstetrician time to come over to the hospital from his office, change, don gown and mask, scrub, and cut the episiotomy without the baby's untimely arrival. Because labor was effectively halted by the spinal, he could deliver the mother when he was prepared, and nurses were less likely to have to catch an early baby. In these situations, the effects on the baby were more pronounced, and there was the probability of decreased oxygen supply to the baby in the last minutes before birth as a result of using spinal anesthesia.

In addition to episiotomy, forceps, and stirrups, the spinal requires for safety that an intravenous drip be placed in the mother's arm, because of the anticipated drop in blood pressure and because the spinal's effect on the uterus' ability to contract may result in excessive bleeding after the birth. The IV drip usually contains Pitocin, a substance to help the uterus contract, and the same substance used to induce or speed labor. Sometimes the woman shivers with cold after delivery because the spinal brings blood to the surface of the body, which cools it, thus dropping the body temperature.

With a spinal, the baby may remain with the parents in the recovery room, and the mother may nurse the baby. Extra care will be required from the husband and the nursing staff until the anesthesia wears off. Usually the mother cannot leave the recovery room until she has regained her ability to urinate. This may require several hours.

Also, she must remain flat for several hours after birth to help prevent the possibility of a spinal headache. The cause of the headache, lasting up to several days, is thought to be leakage of spinal fluid. The use of fine-gauge needles has reduced this possibility, but it can occur.

Spinal anesthesia is often the anesthesia of choice for Cesarean birth because it allows the mother to remain awake. She may, however, prefer an epidural (see below) for a Cesarean.

*Saddle-block anesthesia* is similar to spinal anesthesia, but it numbs only the part of the body that would rest on a saddle. Generally, it is impossible to move one's legs. It is administered in the same way as a spinal, but at a somewhat lower place in the back. A spinal headache is possible, and all other side effects ascribed to the spinal also apply to the saddle block. An IV, forceps, and postpartum Pitocin to contract the uterus are standard with this type of anesthesia.

Spinal and saddle blocks are useful when a baby cannot descend because of position or size and needs to be turned or assisted with forceps. Even then, however, sometimes a pudendal block (local anesthesia) can be used instead. An epidural (described below) may be used for this purpose.

*Epidural anesthesia* is another regional anesthesia that has come into more frequent use within the past ten years. Not all hospitals offer it. Some prefer instead to use the more familiar spinals or, if requested, local anesthesia, since epidural anesthesia is expensive and an anesthesiologist must be continuously available over a period of hours to monitor and regulate it.

At first, the epidural appears to be the nearly ideal anesthesia. This type of anesthesia is similar to the continuous caudal anesthesia but is introduced into a slightly different location in the patient's back. Like the caudal, it does not enter the spinal fluid. Unlike the other regional anesthesias, spinal and saddle block, which are given at the end of the labor, epidurals can be given before transition, the shortest but usually the most painful part of the labor. Epidurals also have the advantage of not producing the temporary paralysis that results from spinal anesthesia. As with spinals, patients remain awake. Pain relief is generally complete, with a failure rate under 3 percent, but occasionally the epidural "takes" on only one side.

The lower back is swabbed with disinfectant and a needle is inserted to a depth of perhaps half an inch into the epidural space below the spinal cord, where there are many nerve endings. (If the anesthesia seeps into the spinal fluid, it becomes an unintentional spinal.) A small plastic tube, called a catheter, is threaded into the needle and placed in her back where it remains. The rest of the length of the tube is then brought up behind the shoulder and taped into place on the chest, where more anesthetizing fluid can be added during the labor as needed.

An intravenous must also be given, first, to help maintain blood pressure and, second, to give medications (such as Pitocin) to stimulate labor contractions, which are diminished by the epidural. Pitocin may slow the fetal heart rate.

Epidurals can be used for pain relief in normal birth. In many hospitals, especially teaching hospitals, they have become almost routine for normal births unless parents object—even for couples who have attended natural childbirth classes. Childbirth instructors suggest in most circumstances that a woman not take any chemical pain relief *in anticipation* of pain, but only if pain actually occurs and is not relieved adequately by walking, going to the bathroom, using pillows, changing position, increasing deep-muscle relaxation, or changing breathing techniques.

Epidurals can even be used for Cesareans and are often chosen as an alternative to spinals for such surgery. As the baby is removed, there may be some sensation of tugging, but not all women find that unpleasant. Also, epidurals are sometimes used when the baby remains in the persistent posterior position, causing more pain than the woman wishes to accept or requiring the use of forceps.

Fatigue, however, may not be a reason to accept an epidural. Fatigue is often a subjective evaluation that reflects doubts or the suggestion of others that one is tired. People not in labor who are told they look tired often feel fatigue they hadn't felt until the suggestion was made. When told they look well, on the other hand, their eyes brighten and they rally. Just because one has been in labor for hours, or a day, may not produce tiredness in the usual sense, especially if the woman was well nourished and well rested during the last weeks of pregnancy. Sometimes, the suggestion of fatigue is made by the doctors and nurses waiting for the birth because the day has been long for them and they want some defined end to the labor.

Women with epidurals must be watched constantly, and their blood pressure must be taken at least every ten minutes because, as with spinals, blood pressure tends to drop suddenly. Unlike spinals, the epidural is in place during labor, often for several hours. Therefore, the baby's heart must also be checked constantly and a fetal heart monitor (Chapter Four) is recommended. Accordingly, the bag of waters must be ruptured artificially to get the most accurate reading with an internal monitor attached to the baby's scalp. The decreased maternal blood pressure and consequent risk of less oxygen available to the baby may be a contraindication to the use of a major regional technique.

With an epidural, the uterus tends to contract less efficiently. The baby's head may therefore remain high, or the baby may not rotate as easily into the normal anterior (face-down-for-delivery) position, thereby increasing the chance of a Cesarean. Also, the woman is immobilized, and although she can move her legs, they are heavy and weak. She cannot walk. She usually remains in a semi-sitting position to keep the anesthetizing fluid low in her body. This immobility also can put stress on the baby, and is an additional reason for using a fetal heart monitor to obtain a continuous recording.

If labor does not progress, or if there are major fluctuations in the fetal heart rate, a Cesarean may be done with no additional anesthesia required. In fact, the routine use of epidural anesthesia has been associated with the increased rate of Cesarean births.

The epidural is stated to have no direct effect on the baby, although it does pass the placenta. A baby born after epidural anesthesia may have slightly reduced muscle tone temporarily but is otherwise alert.

The later in labor the epidural is given, the less opportunity for interfering with the progress of labor and the fetal heart rate. The amount of Xylocaine or Marcane used varies. A light dose near the end of labor may give rise to few or no problems.

With an epidural, the urge to push is inhibited or absent. The woman can still push, although somewhat less effectively because usually she has no feeling in that part of her body. An IV, fetal heart monitor, Pitocin, stirrups, episiotomy, and forceps are the usual accompaniments of epidural anesthesia.

After the birth, the intravenous must remain in place to help contract the uterus with Pitocin. As with other regional anesthesia —the spinal and saddle block—and as with gas anesthesia, there is likely to be more postpartum bleeding than the usually small amount of uterine blood and fluid.

During the time the epidural is in place, the bladder often fills with fluid unnoticed, sometimes interfering with the descent of the baby's head. If the baby is pulled with forceps when the bladder is full, there is the possibility of damaging the bladder and of contracting a postpartum bladder infection. This does occur, although statistics on the frequency are unavailable. Postpartum urinary retention is common with epidurals, and a catheter may be used to drain the bladder after epidural anesthesia. The use of the catheter is associated with increased urinary tract and bladder infections.

GENERAL ANESTHESIA

The general anesthesia formerly in use in the last minutes before the birth was the inhalation (gas) type, mostly ether, often cyclopropane.

Although the figure for maternal mortality at childbirth is exceedingly low, nearing the zero point, anesthesia has been an occasional cause. Since food in the stomachs of women under ether could be vomited then aspirated (causing blockage of the airways and death if resuscitative techniques were not effective), the widespread use of general anesthesia was the original reason that women were made to fast during labor, a requirement that still predominates in the majority of institutions and is only now beginning to change. Gas anesthesia tended to produce blue, sluggish babies.

A lawsuit in 1963 by the husband of a patient who had received general anesthesia and, as a result of an error, died, began the halt to the use of general anesthesia for normal childbirth. For a time it was used in low doses to relax the uterus for the purpose of turning a breech baby for delivery. However, standard medical practice now dictates that breech babies be delivered by Cesarean section. So inhalation anesthesia is generally not used for breech births, either.

General anesthesia is occasionally used for Cesareans, but most informed couples usually request a regional anesthesia block so that the mother will be awake. However, if a spinal cannot be done because of 1) anomalies in the bones of the back or 2) low maternal blood pressure and slowed fetal heart rate, perhaps due to a long labor fast and lying in a supine position, then a "general" might be ordered. Sometimes physicians prefer general anesthesia, since gas can be administered slightly faster than a spinal.

Information on anesthesia used for childbirth is available at all hospitals. U. S. Government figures show that during nearly half of all deliveries nationwide, including Cesareans, anesthesia other than local is used. The other half receive either local or no anesthesia.

# Chapter Four

# HOSPITAL PROCEDURES DURING LABOR

Most couples still give birth in hospitals, although a small but growing number now arrange for out-of-hospital births. This movement has had an effect on the way hospital births are conducted, especially in making available hospital birth rooms for delivery.

## BIRTH ROOMS

Birth rooms are intended to meet the demand for an entirely natural, unmanaged birth without the routine interventions that have become part of so many hospital births. Here women labor and deliver in the same room, which was, until recently, a truly revolutionary concept. Obstetricians, sometimes midwives if available, attend the birth. Parents spend time with their babies in the birth room after delivery, remaining there for an indeterminate length of time, depending largely on how many other laboring patients have requested the room. Parents then go to a room in the postpartum area, perhaps keeping the baby with them. Some are discharged home. Most hospitals now have at least one birth room, and more are being readied to meet the demand for natural childbirth in a homelike setting. Anesthesia is normally not used in birth rooms, and if it is desired, the couple must usually move to a labor or delivery room.

Whereas sometimes the equipment for obstetrical intervention is in the birth room itself, some birth rooms are beautifully flexible to the parents' needs, with shower, a comfortable bed, or even a birth chair or birthing stool. Other children in the family may visit during part or all of the labor. Refreshments are available or may be brought from home to allay the hunger of any member of the family, including the woman giving birth. Obstetricians or midwives may be in attendance at the birth without ceremonial, but often useless, gowns and masks.

Birth rooms may have requirements for their use, which must be checked ahead of time before selecting a hospital. Some labor and delivery units require an appointment with a hospital nurse beforehand so that the staff can ascertain the parents' needs. Some parents may be screened out of the birth room because of medical problems, such as the probability that the birth will be by Cesarean. Sometimes, a couple who delivers too far from the due date may be refused use of the birth room.

Since older women are more likely to have a Cesarean, women over thirty-five (sometimes younger) may be rejected by birthroom policies even if there is no hypertension and if tests during pregnancy have shown no birth defect. Women over thirty-five often have a harder time defending their request for a normal birth, even though there is no reason to anticipate problems. Health status seems to be the important determinant, and this depends on factors such as nutrition, exercise, and stress management. Some persons suggest that almost everyone should be offered the option of a birth room. After all, the mother can be moved if necessary, or needed equipment can be brought in.

## HOSPITAL BIRTH AND HOW IT CAME TO BE

It is difficult for many hospitals today to provide non-interventionist birth, even when the risks of intervention are acknowledged. Reimbursement is determined by procedures done, not those avoided by education and prevention. Professional training and promotional activities on the part of drug and medical equipment companies all act to promote intervention.

In order to understand current hospital procedures, it is necessary to look at the history of maternity care in this country.

The 1946 Hillburton Act provided massive amounts of government money to build hospitals in underserved areas. These hospitals needed indigent women as clinic patients to test new obstetrical and gynecological techniques. In return, these women received free care. In the interest of expanding medical knowledge, new ways of managing birth could be attempted, without requirements from outside governmental agencies, consumer groups, or other health professionals that these new methods were safe. No controlled studies on safety were done before a practice or procedure was introduced. Perhaps the practice was expedient. It might help control infection or meet hospital space and staffing needs. Untested armchair hypotheses were rampant, and untested practices became ritual.

Hospital maternity care, and to a somewhat lesser extent all hospital care, is still based on this charity-patient model. It was the economically or socially disadvantaged women who first came to hospitals to have their babies, the poor women who had no private physician to come to their homes, the unwed mothers who had no homes, and the sick women needing medical treatment. This pattern of care, with few deviations (such as private rooms after delivery), became standard for all patients hospitalized for birth. Gradually, as this medical model of birth became more widespread, physicians began to believe that there was no such thing as a truly "normal" birth.

In the hospitals there was no place for midwives and no training for them. Physicians controlled hospital birth because medical fees were still low and doctors could not afford the competition of midwives. Besides, they needed the indigent population for their own training.

Women had little say in maternity care, whether they were patients or professionals. The cult of female weakness and infirmity continued into this century and was documented in medical texts. In hospitals women were either patients, nurses (who followed doctors' orders), clerical workers, or cleaning women.

Hospital administrators and physicians were at first concerned that the more affluent women would not come to the hospitals. Hospitals had long been viewed as a place to die. Private patients would share common labor rooms and use the same delivery rooms as the charity patients, who were seen as carrying diseases and lice. Furthermore, the hospital routines had evolved to meet the needs of staff. The atmosphere was impersonal and dehumanizing. Patients and their families had little say about any aspect of their care. In fact, women were separated from all family members, including their babies. The care model was that of the industrial assembly line, not one of individualized care.

Women came to the hospitals because they wanted the drugs for pain, as discussed in the previous chapter. Hospital promotional material told women that the hospital was safer and cleaner than their homes. Finally, physicians became unavailable for home care.

During an earlier century, physicians had been concerned that women, for reasons of modesty, would not change from midwives to male physicians. However, the initial objections of women to having males assist at birth was overcome by the fact that the physicians were seen as being of a higher social class. And they cost more. Therefore, before the rise of the hospitals, having a doctor come to one's home to attend at a birth had become a status symbol. A nurse might also be hired to attend the birth, because doctors did not do the caretaking that women had traditionally done. One could not expect the doctor to hold one's hand, do the laundry after the birth, feed the mother, and dress the baby.

Also, male doctors had more tools. They had forceps to shorten labor, which they had brought from Europe after the American Revolution. If the uterus had fallen out of position or a bladder had been damaged in childbirth or the vagina had been torn, these could be repaired through techniques practiced on unanesthetized slave women. (Even so, modesty had required until 1900 that women deliver on their sides keeping their skirts on and facing away from the doctor. The birth was done by feel.) Thus, women were already accustomed to male physicians by the time birth moved to the hospital. Anyway, they hardly knew the difference, since they were drugged for the hospital births.

Childbirth practices in hospitals were affected by the ill-understood theory of contagion. This, along with drugs, contributed to the dehumanization of obstetric care. Even now, when contagion is understood, certain practices continue that make little or no sense, such as draping a woman's legs for delivery with sterile sheets that she may not touch.

The germ theory of disease was not known until nearly 1900.

Before this, childbed fever had been a traditional hazard to child-bearing women. An Austrian physician named Semmelweiss, in the 1840s, had discovered the connection between childbed fever and the practice of the same physicians both delivering babies and performing autopsies, and he recommended that doctors scrub their hands with chloride of lime after autopsies. However, his colleagues did not believe his theory, and he died an outcast from the medical establishment of the times. Later, in the United States, Oliver Wendell Holmes published a treatise showing that mothers who were attended by midwives or who delivered at home were likely to be spared, while, in physician-conducted births, the more intervention that occurred, such as inserting the hands or forceps into the vagina, the more infections resulted. Even in the face of this evidence, however, physicians still resisted the theory. Doctors were gentlemen, and gentlemen, it was reasoned, have clean hands.

In 1927 childbed fever killed 15 percent of the patients in one hospital. It was still a problem until the 1950s and beyond, as hospital "staph" infections tended to become resistant to antibiotics. Even to this day, hospitals and hospital procedures are still a source of infection.

To control disease, a more active management of normal birth was encouraged. Birth was seen as a dangerous event. To clean out the fever, nurses were required to bathe and change uniforms. Wards were aired. The possibility of lice from crowded tenement areas started the practice of sending the patient's clothes home in a paper bag. Women had their pubic hair shaved, and were often washed with kerosene or ether. Enemas became routine, although the connection between enemas and childbed fever was only hypothesized and never clear.

The desire to control infection ran concurrently with the wish to expedite delivery. The amniotic sac was broken to release the waters, the delivery was expedited with forceps, and the expulsion of the placenta was hurried by pushing on the abdomen. These procedures are still done, but the rationale for doing them has changed, as will be described in the following chapters. Sometimes douches of bichloride of mercury were used, too, and the syringes used to give them were not disinfected between patients.

The infections in the crowded institutions housing women, babies, and staff, both the sick and the well, continued. Not until the 1950s did the McBryde study at Duke University show that there were fewer infections in family-centered care units, in which the mother and baby were housed together with the father also allowed in the room, instead of in central nurseries with both mother and baby exposed to a large number of personnel. The old assembly-line model exposed mothers and babies to many people, including hospital staff with colds and other infections.

The fathers were long considered to be a source of infection. This was the ostensible reason why for long years he was limited to waiting rooms, with only short visiting hours with his wife when the baby was in the nursery. Under no circumstance could he touch or even be in the same room with the baby until he took his wife and child home. If the care was bad, the woman had little recourse, since if she left the hospital early with her husband, she had to leave the infant behind because she had no access to the nursery. Also, she knew nothing about umbilical cord care or what to do about her stitches, or how to make formula. She was, in effect, a powerless inmate within the institution.

Siblings could not visit as a result of public health regulations prohibiting visitors under the age of fourteen, in order to minimize communicable disease. The problem of infection also supported the organization of maternity care into a series of separate experiences. (A law remains on the Massachusetts books that prohibits laboring and delivering in the same room. Thus, the origin of the labor room and the separate delivery room to which the patient is transferred minutes before birth. The recent birth rooms are considered legal because they constitute an "experiment.") Labor and delivery nurses were not seen in the postpartum area of the hospital after the birth. Nor did nursery nurses take care of the mother after the birth. Postpartum nurses still do not appear in the labor and delivery unit or in the nursery.

The efficiency of drugs and anesthesia, an emphasis on specialization, and the measures to control infection contributed to the change away from the midwifery style of care. From 1930 to 1960, the transition from home birth to hospital birth was virtually complete. Only recently has the midwifery style of care—

where one person cared for the woman during pregnancy, labor, and delivery, and immediately afterward, including counseling on infant care and breast-feeding—been revived. Providers of maternity care are responding to the needs of parents who have been educated for childbirth.

## WHEN TO GO TO THE HOSPITAL

"I'll be so embarrassed if I don't know false labor from true labor and have to be sent home. Or I'll go to the hospital too soon and wait for hours with nothing really happening. I could even go too late and not make it!"

The assumption is often made that there is a "correct" time to appear at the hospital. Therefore, many parents begin the process of birthing with a distinct loss of self-esteem and feeling of defensiveness. When they arrive, they want reassurance that they came at "the right time."

Obstetricians at busy office prenatal visits often answer this question with a noncommittal, "Oh, you'll know." They may have a hand-out sheet for patients, but unless pressed they most typically do not volunteer much, if any, information about going to the hospital or what to expect when couples get there. Sometimes they say that a couple should go to the hospital when the contractions are five minutes apart if a primipara (a woman having a first delivery) or when the contractions are observable and regular if a multipara (a woman who has previously given birth). However, this is only a rule of thumb because labor patterns differ enormously. Indeed, it is hard to give firm guidelines, since the only fixed pattern in labor is the one-minute length of each contraction and the fact that there will be three stages.

If a couple calls into the obstetrician's office with contractions or with a gush of water, he likely will say, "Come on in to the hospital," even if it is the middle of the night and labor isn't really established. The obstetrician can't be sure what part of labor the woman is in, but the invitation to come on in sounds welcoming. It also has the ring of authority. Because it is hard to know the answer to this apparently ordinary question, the simplest and safest answer is "Come on in"—safe, that is, in terms of getting there on time, but perhaps not in terms of being allowed a normal labor.

Many obstetricians and parents agree that couples enter the hospital far too early, too early not because of the tedium or the cost of the hospital room, but because it can be downright hazardous to mother and child's well-being. Early admission can place decisions in the hands of the hospital staff instead of the parents, and can even lead to an otherwise unnecessary Cesarean birth. So strongly is this recognized that many parents and professionals have proposed that pregnant women labor at home until they reach 6 to 8 centimeters of dilation, attended by one or more women from a cadre of knowledgeable attendants trained in assessing labor progress and checking the basic vital signs of mother and baby.

## THE BEGINNING OF LABOR

Technically, the first stage of labor begins when the cervix begins to dilate, but frequently effacement (flattening, as longitudinal uterine muscles pull the cervix back and circular muscle fibers around the cervix let go) or dilation can be checked manually long before any contractions are noticed. Women may walk around for a week with a dilation fo 4 centimeters even. The Braxton Hicks or practice contractions, known sometimes as "false labor," begin to do the work of labor and in that sense are not "false" at all. Sometimes contractions are occurring, but are not strong enough to awaken the mother, with the result that she gets up in the morning with significant labor progress, causing her to think that her labor is very short.

The mechanism that starts labor at a particular time is not entirely understood, but it is known that the distention of the uterus and the beginning dilation of the cervix, aided by the Braxton Hicks contractions, lead to increased production of oxytocin by the pituitary gland. The oxytocin then encourages further contractions of the uterus.

The woman does not know the degree of dilation, whether 2, 5, or 8 centimeters, since the dilating cervix produces no sensations. And even if she did know, predictions are virtually worthless. She may stay at a certain degree of dilation for hours, or a few contractions may do the whole job, bringing her right up to 10 centimeters and ready to do second-stage pushing. Some women work into labor slowly, having on-again-off-again labor over several days and then progress quickly to 10 centimeters. Occasionally, labor does not progress and the head remains high for a particular reason; for example, if the pelvis is not large enough to accommodate the baby. Every labor is different.

Childbirth is more art than science. A medical professional can only gather information and observe the individual situation with input from the woman and those who are with her.

Couples often prefer a slow, intermittent labor to a rapid, tumultuous and more painful one where everything happens so fast that there is no time to make judgments and exercise options. Some labors are both fast and easy. However, sometimes labors that stop for no apparent reason or do not progress at the arbitrary medical standard of 1 centimeter per hour produce anxiety and guilt in the couple. Everyone is waiting for "progress," a word with heavy psychological impact, and the new parents may dislike to keep those around them waiting.

Increased knowledge can diminish the almost phobic fear of "not making it" to the sometimes illusory safety of the hospital. It is only common sense to keep in touch with the whereabouts of one's spouse and to notify the obstetrician or midwife, and any other labor-support people, that labor appears imminent and that another call can be expected. Then, if the woman, with her mate, attempts to feel in touch with and assess the pattern and strength of the contractions, she can feel some sense of control. Sometimes contractions begin in her back, then radiate around to the front. For some, they may remain in the back during much of the labor. The appearance of the mucous plug or "bloody show" may indicate that labor is imminent, or it may be a couple of days hence. An occasional woman has a two- or three-contraction labor such as described in a newspaper headline, "Fagan [the father] delivers fast fifth [baby]." In most cases, parents need not fear an unexpected birth. The woman may at times delay the birth up to half an hour by doing her "don't push" breathing. The alternative to this sort of uncertainty is to induce the baby on a selected date and hold off the baby's arrival with a spinal until the doctor gets there to deliver it. The paradox in the past has been that those with fast, easy labors are most likely to have subsequent babies induced and delivered with regional anesthesia. Those living an hour or more from the hospital may face the same dilemma, whether to "take a chance" or have an induced labor.

In actuality, the same doubts and crisis orientation occur within the hospital. When should the doctor be called? If he is called too soon away from his office full of prenatal and gynecological patients, he may be angry. This is a problem the midwifery model helps to resolve, since the midwife has the advantage of being already in the hospital providing labor care as well as delivery care. She is there when needed, without having to be called.

Many people, including hospital staff, tend to measure the length of the labor as the time between arrival at the hospital and the birth, somehow seeing labor at home as not really labor. The occasional contractions at work that day or during the preceding night are largely ignored, and the measured time doesn't begin until the patient is ensconced on the turf of the medical establishment and the labor record begins to be charted. When couples come into the hospital later in labor, as is becoming the custom in many places, both staff and parents come to expect shorter labors. When the length of labor stretches to ten or twelve hours, even for a first-time mother, worried "hurry-up" messages are conveyed to the parents.

Women who have been in the hospital less than ten hours with regular contractions and steady progress, meaning slow dilation at first as is a typical pattern, have heard discussions of a possible C-section with no indication other than length of labor. The "failure to progress" notation made on the chart is the most common reason for a Cesarean birth today, which is why understanding labor progress has become so important. There is no clear line of when labor is too long. When is an obstetrician justified in performing surgery to end the labor? Does the standard goal of 1 centimeter of dilation per hour take into account the array of individual labor patterns? Will parents accept a Cesarean based on this progress requirement even though no one accepts it as dogma?

## THE BREAKING OF THE WATERS AND THE IMPLICATIONS OF RUPTURED MEMBRANES

The breaking of the amniotic sac is a typical first sign of approaching labor. (It's a good idea to place a plastic shower curtain over your mattress during the last month of pregnancy to protect your bed.) Sometimes only the mucous plug appears, dislodged from the cervix by unfelt contractions. Sometimes what appears to be the mucous plug is only the extra vaginal lubrications associated with the approach of labor. Sometimes the fluid is indeed the amniotic fluid beginning as a slow leak. If the leak is very slow, the sac may seal itself up, in which case no more fluid will appear. Or the waters may break in a big, warm gush so sudden that some women actually report hearing or feeling the sac pop like a cork out of a bottle. The amount may be as much as a quart, or so little that there is genuine doubt that the waters have actually broken. At the birth, more of the waters may accompany the arrival of the baby. The fluid continues to be produced even if the sac is no longer intact so that "dry" births do not occur.

Within six to eight hours after the membrane breaks, three quarters of all women will go into active labor. The rest will take longer. Decisions about medical intervention to induce labor may have to be made because it has become standard procedure to deliver the baby within twenty-four or forty-eight hours after the membranes have ruptured, since, without the sac to protect it, the previously sterile area is now open to bacteria and the possibility of infection.

### Amniotomy

If the membranes are ruptured by hospital staff as a method of inducing or speeding labor (or because that is the routine practice of the obstetrician), the procedure is called an amniotomy. The amniotomy is done by inserting a white plastic amnihook, similar to a crochet hook, into the vagina to nick the membrane. No pain is involved, and the woman may be unaware that anything other than an internal exam is occurring unless she or her mate is watching closely. The membrane may also be nicked by a fingernail during an exam and the labor process initiated or speeded either on purpose or inadvertently.

One woman told me:

"I had a Friday afternoon appointment. Because I was near my due date I had an internal exam. My doctor said he'd probably see me tonight in the hospital, and I wondered how he knew. Sure enough, labor started within a few hours. Later I learned that he had nicked the membrane during the exam to induce labor."

Although it is known that infections can occur if there is "unreasonable" delay in delivering the infant after an amniotomy, there are little or no firm data on this subject. There have been cases of lung infections in newborns after prolonged rupture of the membranes. Women's health and home-birth advocates first illuminated the following facts. The possibility of infection is increased by the number and frequency of vaginal exams during labor. At an earlier time vaginal exams during labor were not done; rectal exams were done instead, and the edges of the cervix palpated through the rectal wall. For the past twenty or so years physicians and nurses have preferred vaginal exams, since they allow a more accurate assessment. Sexual intercourse after the membranes have ruptured increases the risk of infection. Sometimes couples use sexual activity, either intercourse or, if the waters have broken, nipple stimulation, in an attempt to stimulate the woman's body production of pitocin and thus initiate labor contractions. Tub baths taken after the membranes are no longer intact may increase the infection risk, too. One case of newborn pneumonia was ascribed to a bubble bath taken during labor. Examining fingers, even covered by a sterile glove, or any object inserted into the vagina, tend to push the normal vaginal flora up into the uterus as well as introduce new ones. For this reason, tampons should not be used to absorb water or "show."

Therefore, a woman whose membranes rupture spontaneously and who plans on a non-interventionist birth, whether at a hospital, birth center, or at home, should be careful not to be overly curious about the degree of cervical dilation, in case labor does not begin or the progress is slow or intermittent. If labor does not begin within two days, she should take her temperature periodically, since a fever could indicate an infection. Obstetricians usually want patients in the hospital once the membranes have broken, but remaining in the hospital for a long stretch of time adds to the risk because of the virulence of hospital bacteria. Also, vaginal exams will be done in the hospital unless the couple explain their wish to reduce the possibility of infection.

If the pregnancy is only seven or so months along and the membrane ruptures spontaneously, the parents and obstetrician have a dilemma. In this case there is usually an attempt to prolong the pregnancy until there is assurance through tests that the infant's lungs are mature enough to allow survival outside of the uterus. At times, alcohol has been taken intravenously to help prevent labor and more recently a drug Ritadine for this purpose has been approved by the Food and Drug Administration.

It is unfortunate that such a normal beginning of labor, the spontaneous breaking of the waters, can have such enormous implications in the hospital's management of the labor and birth that it comes to be seen as an abnormal occurrence. Yet if it does not occur normally, an amniotomy is done. Thus, if a woman is not already defined as high risk because her waters have broken, the hospital staff feels compelled to do the amniotomy and put her at high risk (as they see it). Concerned obstetricians, nurse-midwives, and staffs of alternative birth centers tend to counsel patience, careful watching, avoidance of unnecessary risk factors, and careful assessment of possible intervention.

Other women who call their obstetrician to report that their waters have broken will be admonished, with a sense of urgency, to come to the hospital immediately, and from the moment of hospital admission an arbitrary time limit for giving birth may be proffered by all personnel with whom the couple comes in contact, heralding the fact that someone else will take over if the parents cannot bring forth their young within twenty-four, forty-eight, or occasionally even twelve, hours.

No one really knows how long the labor should continue after the membranes have ruptured, but in the opinion of many, twenty-four hours is too short. To ensure delivery within twenty-four hours after the membrane ruptures, some hospitals administer Pitocin to stimulate labor.

What can happen once the membrane has ruptured? A labyrinth of procedures is likely to await the couple anticipating a normal, natural childbirth. All of them have become "accepted standard procedure," meaning that health professionals tend not to question them and the resulting problems may be perceived as unavoidable. (This does not mean that all obstetricians agree with this stance, though. Some say, unofficially, "I tell my patients who come too early to go back to sleep and call me in the morning.")

First, walking may be prohibited with ruptured membranes, since, without the cushioning effect of the waters, the cord could conceivably become compressed and thus deprive the baby of oxygen. The fallacy, however, is that walking is not prohibited before arriving at the hospital, only after admission to the labor floor. The woman is considered capable to make arrangements to come to the hospital, and to walk to her room. But if she tries to get up to go to the bathroom, she bumps up against the alleged hospital regulation "No ambulation after the membranes break." The fact is that if the baby's head is engaged in the pelvis, the cord can no longer get in a position to be compressed, whatever the mother's position. However, prohibition against walking can adversely affect maternal circulation and the amount of oxygen to the baby. It can slow the progress of labor and increase pain. Also, being bedridden makes it harder for the mother to empty her bladder, especially if she cannot use the bedpan.

Second, if labor does not begin soon after the membranes are ruptured, the woman may be induced by means of the controversial drug Pitocin, the synthesized version of human oxytoxic hormone. Pitocin's effects on labor can be dramatic whether used to induce labor or augment labor already in progress.

"I use Pitocin if her waters break. That may prevent her from getting a Cesarean later," states one of many obstetricians. He does have a point. If he doesn't do all he can to help her dilate, her time allotted for labor (twenty-four hours or even forty-eight), may run out and a Cesarean may be done.

On the other hand, the use of Pitocin can affect the baby's oxygen supply and heart rate, possibly adding an otherwise unnecessary Cesarean to the hospital's statistics. Because of the additional risk, a fetal heart monitor will be attached. The use of

Pitocin, then, will change a labor from the category of normal to that of potentially high risk—if the amniotomy has not already put it in that category. In any event, the use of Pitocin will definitely increase labor pain, so that medication or an epidural may be required. Pitocin will be further discussed later, under "Induced Labor and Laboratory Tests that May Affect Induction Decisions."

Once the membranes are ruptured, if the cervix will not dilate within the prescribed time, or if the measures taken to force dilation are ineffective, a Cesarean will be the medical decision.

Ruptured membranes can take on mammoth significance for the rest of the labor. Amniotomy, especially early in labor before 5 centimeters' dilation, automatically places a woman in a high-risk category for Cesarean section. Hospital policies and routine amniotomies give prospective parents one more reason to fear too-early admission.

A strong reason for not allowing an amniotomy is research indicating that the cushioning waters may provide protection for the baby's head. Dr. Caldeyro-Barcia of the Latin American Center of Perinatology and Human Development in Montevideo, Uruguay, was the first to question the value of the amniotomy. For 66 percent of women, membranes rupture spontaneously at the end of the first stage of labor. Early rupture of the membranes was found to produce shortened labor, disalignment of the fetal cranial bones at birth, possible brain lesions, dips in the fetal heart rate (other than the normal dips associated with contractions), possible compression of the umbilical cord, and increased acidity of the fetal scalp blood at birth.

In certain cases, however, there are sound reasons for an amniotomy. If there are dips in the fetal heart rate (normally 140 plus or minus 10 or more beats per minute), which is where the heart rate does not recover its normal rate immediately after a contraction, or variable dips lasting more than 40 seconds, which could indicate lack of oxygen to the baby, then an amniotomy might be done. This is because, under these conditions it is important to see whether the waters show meconium from the infant's intestines, which along with the slowed heart rate, may indicate fetal distress. The pH of the fetal scalp blood can then be checked by taking a sample during labor. A Cesarean may be indicated.

Sometimes when labor is well established or has been, perhaps, truly long (although this is not easy to define), it may make sense to nick the membrane to encourage the woman to deliver. There are not specific guideposts for this. Birth is as much art as it is science.

By the way, the membranes need never break at all, in which case the baby would be born with a "caul," inside the sac as kittens and certain other mammals. In this case, which is rare, the sac would be broken immediately after birth to permit the baby to draw his first breath.


# INDUCED LABOR
# AND LABORATORY TESTS
# THAT MAY AFFECT INDUCTION DECISIONS:

## "Early Babies, Late Babies"

Some babies need to be induced for medical reasons. One is toxemia, a condition relating to maternal kidney function, which is not entirely understood but is thought to have some relationship to diet, especially to inadequate protein consumption. It is diagnosed by urine tests, which show protein in the urine, and a rise in blood pressure; perhaps also blurred vision and an unusual degree of fluid retention. A Cesarean may be done if immediate delivery is medically indicated.

Diabetic women are often induced because their babies tend to be late and also because of the need for monitoring the infant's insulin level as it makes the transition from intrauterine life in a diabetic woman taking insulin injections. In addition, a true diagnosis of post-maturity and placental insufficiency may be made. The baby could have such a long gestational life that the placenta has begun to "age," or for some other reason the placenta is no longer functioning adequately.

In general, a baby may be expected to arrive within two to three weeks of the calculated due date. However, as described in

Chapter One, there are factors that would make the due date uncertain even if every baby arrived after an exact number of days of fetal development. For example, irregular menstrual cycles and uncertain ovulation often occur after using the birth-control pill. In addition, nursing a previous baby acts to inhibit ovulation (although this is not a reliable contraceptive method), and therefore the time of conception may be uncertain.

Elective inductions done without medical reason have long been recognized by the American College of Obstetrics and Gynecology and by consumer-education groups as increasing babies' risks of lung and respiratory problems. Low-birth-weight babies are also an increased possibility with this procedure.

The federal government's funding of research on induction has been limited. Because Pitocin and Syntocinon which are oxytoxic labor stimulants similar to the body's own labor-stimulating hormone, have been on the market since before 1938, they are exempted under the grandfather clause from Food and Drug Administration regulation. In 1977 the FDA recommended that physicians stop performing elective inductions, primarily because of the undefined benefit-to-risk ratio in relation to these drugs.

The research studies reviewed by the FDA described a slightly increased risk of prematurity, respiratory distress after birth, fetal distress during labor, and jaundice associated with the use of Pitocin and Syntocinon.

The first surgical induction of labor by rupturing the membranes was done in 1609 in France. In 1810, this method was first used in the United States. During World War II, the growing demand for obstetrical services brought a shortage of professional personnel. Overworked obstetricians preferred inductions to help stabilize their unpredictable lives. It was a convenience for doctor and patient alike.

No accurate figures are available for the number of inductions still performed in this country today. The rate has probably declined slightly in the past ten or twelve years, and now most likely approximates 11 percent of all labors. There are regional differences, with rates appearing to be highest in the northeast. Elective inductions have been criticized so severely that the former practice of choosing the baby's birthdate has become outmoded.

## Laboratory Tests to Assess
## the Need for Induction of Labor

There are tests that can help determine the size of the baby during pregnancy and whether it is medically "early" or "late." Some of the tests are invasive as, for example, X rays and laboratory tests involving dyes or catheters; some are non-invasive as, for example, an ultrasound or blood pressure reading, and involve essentially no risk.

The fact that these tests may determine the need for induction of labor or indicate that something is wrong, tends to intimidate many parents. If these tests should become routine for all pregnant women, the problems might outweigh the benefits. However, the tests do diagnose problems and have a definite place in the practice of obstetrics, even though the trips to the hospital during pregnancy for testing tend to increase dependence on the medical staff and concomitantly decrease the parents' trust of their normal body functioning. The tests certainly tend to make parents feel more vulnerable to the dictates of the hospital when they are admitted and, of course, drive up the costs of maternity care.

Yet, obstetricians feel safer when the tests are done. They also feel less vulnerable if they induce a baby too soon than if they do nothing and the baby is truly "late." The test on urine to determine hormone levels is a relatively simple, inexpensive, non-invasive procedure described below. But other tests include late amniocentesis to assess lung maturity and ultrasound to assess growth. The size of the baby as shown by ultrasound is not definitive at this late stage when weight gain rather than bony growth is occurring. Ultrasound is also needed before doing a late pregnancy amniocentesis requiring the woman to go to the hospital. Both of these procedures are described below. They can be overutilized with no real benefit for normal women and infants except to help protect against inducing an immature infant if induction is contemplated.

What makes decisions for parents difficult is that the obstetrician may not recognize from either the tests or manual exploration of the pelvic bone structure, that a baby two or more weeks "late" may grow to a size that the pelvis cannot accommodate.

If the labor does not progress at a reasonable rate, the assumption may be made that the baby is too large because it is late. A "late" baby may then justify a Cesarean delivery. Therefore, the reasoning can run, "An induction now may prevent a Cesarean later." Sometimes, however, the baby is not as large as expected —may even be underweight.

The expectation of a baby "too large" may reduce the length of time labor is "allowed" because if there is surgery to be done, the obstetrician would rather do it as soon as possible. The mother may be told that it is better to do it before she gets too "tired." She may even be told she is "not yet in active labor." If she is uncertain and anxious, and has been allowed nothing to eat or drink for a number of hours, she can easily fear that her strength will not endure.

In inductions there is the possibility that even a cervix that appears "ripe" may not dilate. The use of Pitocin to prod its progress may affect the baby's heart rate adversely, with the result that a Cesarean may be done for fetal distress.

Parents need to use every facet of intelligence and judgment and to utilize information from medical practitioners as wisely as possible during the entire childbearing experience. Couples see childbearing from a special perspective—with their own values, and with a sense of continuity unmatched by providers (although midwives may come close).

Obstetricians are not uncaring, but their viewpoint is toward getting the baby out at a relatively predictable time with no observable problems. Obstetricians, to some extent, must typically define problems differently from informed parents. Obstetricians are most sensitive to possible problems, including legal problems, that could arise out of not acting to intervene in standard ways. They may be uncomfortable, angry, and even frightened by women who walk around for hours with ruptured membranes. If there should be a subsequent rise in maternal temperature or a compressed umbilical cord, it is cause for alarm, and he could be criticized by hospital committees. In the same way, a birth defect that could have been detected during pregnancy by a test, even if the patient refused the test, is an unforgettable experience for the obstetrician. Doing anything differently from the standards accepted by his colleagues can produce an extraordinary degree of stress for the physician.

Parents cannot ignore these factors. But they are also sensitive to emotional factors and long-term developmental factors, intellectual, social, and physical. They are concerned about possible problems relating to intervention as, for example, a Cesarean done supposedly at term that actually turns out to be premature, resulting in a five-pound (or less) baby that perhaps requires special intensive care. Parents are alert to every inkling of expediency replacing patience and time.

The obstetrician is less bothered by problems that result from honest mistakes and currently accepted standards of care, even though these practices may be disavowed in future years. Obstetricians and hospitals have been found not liable by courts if an honest mistake was made or if accepted standards of the time were employed in treatment, even if that treatment results in an adverse outcome. For these reasons, dialogue between parents and health-care providers is essential.

Some of the tests done before hospital admission that may affect the time admission and the possible induction of labor are summarized below:

a) *Ultrasound Test.* High-frequency sound waves are bounced against the maternal abdomen, giving a two-dimensional outline of the fetus. This may be done in mid-pregnancy to ascertain fetal size for help in pinpointing the due date. If the baby is "small for dates," the due date may be moved ahead.

Ultrasound can also help determine the position of the baby and the location of the placenta. The parents can watch the baby move as reflected on the screen and take home a picture.

Some parents refuse this test if there is no specific medical reason for it. The safety of ultrasound is not yet definitely determined, but the assumption of relative safety is made. In any case, it is safer than X ray. Animal experiments have shown that neurological damage can result from "excessive" use of ultrasound, but effects in human infants can be difficult to determine. The Food and Drug Administration currently withholds judgment until further research is done. (The safety of fetal heart monitors during labor, however, is being questioned, because these monitors also work on the principle of ultrasound, and remain in place on the abdomen for many hours.

The activity of the baby may be observed by its response to sound. The laboratory worker may bang on pans to make noise and then observe the fetal movement and increased heart rate response by ultrasound. Activity of the fetus is then positively correlated with health. Sometimes the child's sex, prior to birth, can be observed in the ultrasound "picture."

Ultrasound equipment is now being purchased by some obstetrical practices for use in their offices to monitor fetal growth throughout pregnancy.

**b)** *Amniocentesis* is the well-publicized test that can detect Down's Syndrome, a form of mental retardation formerly known as mongoloidism. This and other chromosomal disorders, including neural tube defects such as spinal bifida, are diagnosed by analyzing cells in the fetal amniotic fluid, which is drawn from the amniotic sac by syringe. An ultrasound test is done prior to the amniocentesis to locate the baby and placenta for proper insertion of the needle, although the baby would naturally move out of the way anyway.

The test is done between the fourteenth and sixteenth week of pregnancy, with results available three weeks later, after the cells have been cultured. This chromosomal test also reveals the sex of the fetus, although some parents request that they not be informed of this before the birth.

Since the incidence of Down's Syndrome increases rapidly with maternal age (a woman aged forty-five has a one-in-forty chance of this chromosomal disorder, while for a woman between forty and forty-five it is one per hundred, and for a woman under thirty the odds are one in 1,500), this test is sometimes recommended for older mothers. In fact, physicians who have not informed prospective parents of the availability of amniocentesis and compared for them the risk of amniocentesis with the risk of having a child with a genetic defect have been found legally liable.

Many older parents can find the test valuable, in that it reassures them that their baby will not have Down's Syndrome. During late pregnancy fetal lung maturity can also be measured with this technique, if an induced delivery or a Cesarean is being contemplated. In this case the test determines the L/S (lecithin/sphyngomyelin) ratio which indicates lung maturity. If induction is contemplated because the waters have been broken for an extended time or for some other reason and the lungs are not mature, they can be made so by administering corticosteroids which inhibit lung cell division and encourages lung cells to mature. There is still much that is not known about the use of this procedure. Optimum dosages have not been determined nor have long-term risks been evaluated.

The risks of amniocentesis to the mother are trauma, hemorrhage, and infection. The risks for the fetus are the same. The penetration of the needle through the uterus can produce bleeding. Previous extensive pelvic surgery or infections increase these risks.

Data on subsequent effects of the test are being studied. Many physicians feel that amniocentesis slightly increases the risk of premature rupture of membranes and miscarriage. For this reason, if a baby is conceived after years of infertility or near the end of the childbearing years, the couple may wish to forego amniocentesis. If the couple will not consider an abortion even if a chromosomal defect is discovered, the test serves little purpose.

c) *Stress Test.* During late pregnancy, the woman is sometimes admitted to the hospital and hooked up to a fetal monitor while Pitocin is dripped into her arm intravenously to produce a series of uterine contractions. If the fetal heart "holds up," the infant is adjudged in good condition. The purpose of this test is to assure that "late" babies are still getting adequate oxygen through the placenta and are not post-mature. Sometimes an induced labor results. Many have criticized this procedure, and it is becoming less common.

d) *The Non-stress Test.* Here the fetal heart rate and fetal movements are monitored *without* the use of Pitocin. The purpose of this test is to determine that the baby is in good condition and does not require immediate delivery. When done as a routine test it may mean an extra trip to the hospital and be a source of unnecessary concern.

e) *Estriol Tests* may be done on maternal urine to measure

levels of hormonal estriol, which gives information on possible post-maturity. This is a simple, non-invasive test repeated at intervals.


## ADMISSION PROCEDURES

**a)** *The First Twenty Minutes.* Entering the hospital is a momentous event. The mood may be jocular, hopeful, excited, fearful, uncertain, or a combination of all. This may be the woman's first admission ever. Couples are emotionally as well as physically vulnerable to what lies ahead, and they will always remember what happens.

The first twenty minutes after admission can exert a strong influence on the entire childbirth experience. The husband's presence and participation are critical. He should not be parking the car or filling out admission forms (often some of the paperwork can be done ahead of time). Many decisions are made in the first twenty minutes. Hospital staff may encourage well-intentioned "coffee breaks" for the support people, including husbands. However, in practice this can result in a discontinuity similar to that of the traditional hospital-care model. During this time there is little predictability about relationships with staff, and there are decisions to be made about the labor itself.

> "She couldn't take a coffee break so why should I?" asked a new father. "I knew I was needed. A friend of mine left to call his office and by the time he got back they had started an induction on his wife which neither of them had wanted. He wasn't there to discuss it. Anyway, it was like a movie. No matter how long it might be I wasn't intending to leave in the middle."

During the first twenty minutes, the decision may be made about the availability and appropriateness of a birth room instead of the traditional labor room. (Sometimes a later move can be made when there is a birth room available, but the avoidance of moving from one place to another during labor is one purpose of birth rooms.) Because birth-room facilities are few and cannot usually be reserved but are assigned on a first-come first-served basis, sometimes couples come to the hospital early in labor to get a birth room, or call ahead to make sure one is available before being admitted.

**b)** *Relationships with Staff and Suggestions for Parents.* Progress has been made in many hospitals, allowing a sensitive welcoming and supportive approach uncommon only a few years ago. Both parents, not only the woman, usually prefer a nurturing not patronizing or aggressive approach, although couples can be misled into perceiving coercive, aggressive hospital staff as somehow providing better care. Other couples do not wish to fight the hospital in areas of disagreement, preferring not to detract from the joy of the birth itself.

Couples and staff gauge each other early in the labor, taking the other's measure. What do the couples know? What do they want? Do they really mean what they say or is it intended just as a guide? The parents wish to meet the staff and find out what to expect. They may have already toured the facility and talked with the staff during the pregnancy. Occasionally couples unhappy with an adverse relationship at one hospital have even left during labor to deliver elsewhere. A visit prior to labor can help to avoid this eventuality.

The institutional structure gives the appearance of being heavily weighted in favor of medical providers. Couples are giving birth in unfamiliar surroundings. Other persons with designated responsibilities appear to make all decisions. The obstetricians have been trained to believe that increased intervention will mean a "better" baby, and feel more secure if all the weapons in the medical armamentarium are used despite corresponding risks. However, the hospital's authority is not unlimited. Although patients cannot demand services the hospital does not provide, they can, if worse comes to worse, refuse procedures.

**c)** *Consent Forms and Hospital Admission.* The blanket consent form is presented for signature at the time of admission to absolve the hospital for unanticipated results of treatment. It allows the hospital to give whatever treatment is deemed necessary. In actuality, the prospective patients have not signed away their rights, although many think they have. The effect of the form is more psychological than legally binding.

In the event of an unfavorable outcome, physicians are not protected by the form. Both physicians and lawyers admit that the blanket consent form is not worth the paper it is written on. Patients may cross out parts of it or add sentences to it or not sign it at all. Or later they may repudiate what they did sign, preferring to sign for each procedure individually. If a Cesarean is contemplated, they can expect to be given another consent form to sign.

## The "Prep" and Enema

The "prep" (the shaving of the pubic hair) and enema are two standard admission procedures. They do not affect the course of the labor as does artificial rupture of the membranes. Their purpose is to prepare the birth area.

Nevertheless, these procedures can be distressing and unnecessary despite their long acceptance as one of the rituals of birth. The question "Why" was long obscured by "Why not?" Now that they are usually presented as options, however, both procedures are fast disappearing, especially the enema.

### THE PREP

The ostensible reasons for the prep are: 1) The obstetricians prefer it. 2) Hair harbors germs. 3) There might be a Cesarean and it is good to be ready just in case. 4) It is needed for the episiotomy. 5) Why not?

The reasons advanced against it are: 1) It's demeaning and unnecessary. 2) The hair itches when it grows back. 3) A research study shows that infections are more likely with a prep than without because of razor nicks. 4) Routine episiotomies are probably not a good idea, anyway. 5) Hair around the vagina is usually minimal, so why shave the whole pubic area in case of an episiotomy? Excessive "treatment" based on contingencies may be compared with shoveling the snow before it falls, says a physician expert on iatrogenic, or physician-induced, illness.

A typical compromise is a "miniprep" or "poodle cut" in which only the hair in the area of a possible episiotomy is shaved. The woman may prefer to do it herself before she comes to the hospital.

THE ENEMA

Historically, enemas were associated with health even if birth or surgery were not contemplated. If the patients were to be unconscious or unfit for a day or so, it seemed only sensible to "clean them out" ahead of time, whatever the problem. At one time, enemas were also thought to reduce the hazard of childbed fever.

The reasons still given for the enema are: 1) It stimulates the uterus to contract (which it does). 2) An empty rectum gives more room for the baby. 3) When the woman pushes for the delivery she may involuntarily empty the rectum. 4) The sore episiotomy incision will make it difficult to empty the rectum for a few days after the birth. 5) Why not?

The reasons offered against it are: 1) It should be the woman's decision. She will know if she is constipated. 2) Diarrhea, not constipation, is common the day or two preceding the onset of labor. 3) Enemas are dehumanizing. 4) A woman given an enema may become fearful of eating early in labor, erroneously assuming this will fill the rectum during labor. 5) It is surprisingly uncommon that a woman will push out feces with the baby. Even if it does occur, it is unimportant and hardly noticeable, and is easily whisked away by the nurses. In fact, if this does happen, it is easier to take care of solid material than the watery remains of an enema.

## Do We Have to Have a Fetal Heart Monitor?

"Do we have to's" and "are we allowed to's" pepper the discussions of expectant parents in childbirth classes. The questions might be better framed, "Should we request—?" or "Is it desirable to have—?" and "What are the advantages of—?"

A few years ago electronic fetal heart monitors were only a spot on the horizon. Dr. Edward Hon of Connecticut developed a product and formed the first company to market it, but the new product was not readily accepted until a government grant was given to two hospitals for study of the new device. The hospitals welcomed the award, assuring concerned consumer groups that the monitors would not be used on the natural childbirth women, but on high-risk patients only.

By 1975, however, fetal heart monitors had come into general use, the theory being that *every* woman is potentially high risk. Consumer health groups and obstetricians could not agree on standards for their use. Once the machines were in place in the labor and delivery units, and the company salesmen had trained the staff to use them, the inevitable result was a trend toward using them on everyone. Monitors were accordingly purchased in greater quantity. The machines are expensive, each costing several thousand dollars depending on the model, but the equipment generates revenue for the hospital, because monitoring is billable to insurance companies. Many parents with insurance are unaware of these costs, which affect them only indirectly. The national cost of electronic fetal monitoring was $300 million in 1980.

Also, in many hospitals the monitors have doubled the number of C-sections performed, which, in turn, has increased the incidence of respiratory distress syndrome, a possible consequence of Cesarean birth. Although the monitor can decrease infant mortality slightly, this improvement is seen only among high-risk patients. As a result of a government study on routine electronic monitoring, this practice is beginning to fall out of favor.

With the monitor, a record of every fetal heartbeat can be preserved, along with a record of the contractions and the mother's heartbeat. The companies selling the monitors state that this monitor tape can protect the physician and the hospital against possible malpractice suits. However, this record could also work the other way: If the tape does not show justification for surgery, the physician might be liable for performing an unnecessary Cesarean.

Parents are often surprised by the equipment. Their first knowledge of it may come when they are admitted to the hospital, but socialized to accept enigmas of the hospital, many take the equipment in stride as a new way to assure safety. Other parents are outraged, however, seeing the equipment as a trespass that may even lead to an otherwise unnecessary Cesarean birth.

Obstetricians and hospital personnel may express wonder that their judgment is questioned. For them there is no problem. What can be measured should be measured. But many doctors have backed off from routine monitoring. Other obstetricians still say, "If I don't use a monitor, my colleagues give me a hard time. The nurses don't understand. I feel like a maverick." Electronic fetal monitoring is one of the procedures that tends to diminish the parents' control over the birth, sometimes directly, sometimes subtly. Typically, prepared parents express the need for knowledge that will allow them to "stay in control." Many health professionals also feel this need to maintain control, despite changing relationships between patients and professionals. These physicians feel that it is their charge to manage birth, to take decisive action in the manner of a general commanding his troops. This is their job, and they know more than the patients. The patient's role is to trust and obey. This is the unwritten covenant. But productive discussions can occur despite the differing viewpoints. Monitors do, after all, have a place in obstetrical care.

## Types of Fetal Monitoring Equipment

There are two major types of monitors: *external* and *internal*. Either or both may be used during a labor. Both, looking like large black boxes about two feet long with dials, are wheeled into the room on a metal stand. At times there is no word of explanation other than, "It's so we can listen to your baby," as the hospital staff sets about attaching the patient to the machine. The ambiance is that of an intensive-care unit, where heart attack victims, accident cases, and serious postoperative patients are placed. The couple's excitement on the day to be ever after celebrated as their child's birthday generally takes on a sober if not somber note as the equipment arrives and is attached. Conversation stops. Attention focuses on the black box beside the bed and the high-pitched, continuous beeping sound usually emanating from it.

### EXTERNAL FETAL HEART MONITOR

This type of monitor uses continuous ultrasound. Gel may be placed on the woman's abdomen to provide contact for electronic leads, and a black belt placed around her abdomen. The baby's heart rate, and perhaps also the mother's, will be recorded digitally in flashing numbers on the black box and on slowly unrolling graph paper. The frequency and approximate strength of contractions may be recorded from the changes in pressure on the measuring instrument from the abdomen.

Although the equipment varies to some degree from model to model, it always involves a recording instrument on a table next to the bed and an external attachment to the woman's abdomen. The gel substance facilitates transmission of sound waves, which are produced by a transducer and echoed back. The high-frequency sound waves are converted into signals that can be observed on an oscilloscope or recorded photographically on tape. This equipment replaces listening directly to the baby's heartbeat with a fetascope, similar to the familiar stethoscope. Sometimes it also replaces both the doctor's palpating the uterus to check frequency and strength of contractions and the woman's own report of her contractions. The continuous reading during the entire labor usually is recorded on a strip of paper several yards long which slowly unrolls throughout the labor.

ADVANTAGES

**a)** If the fetal heart rate slows or stops, or if it is slow to recover from the normal slight deceleration during a contraction, this will be apparent.

**b)** No equipment is placed inside the woman's body, or attached directly to the baby. This type of monitor is non-invasive.

**c)** If the heartbeat is difficult to hear with the fetascope because of, for example, maternal obesity, the monitor will be able to pick it up.

**d)** Toxemia, a premature labor, a diabetic mother, or previous uterine surgery make the monitor a helpful tool indeed. If meconium, a tarry substance from the fetal intestines, appears during labor instead of soon after birth, this potential problem may indicate the need for a monitor.

**e)** Possible cord compression, resulting perhaps from long-ruptured membranes or the baby's head not being engaged within the pelvis, and subsequent oxygen deprivation to the baby can be detected. Also, an unfavorable result from induced labor or the use of Pitocin to speed labor can be observed with the monitor. The use of epidural anesthesia usually requires the need for monitoring.

f) Some parents feel reassured by the rhythmic beating of the baby's heart.

g) Nurses can check the woman at intervals longer than fifteen minutes, the usual interval between fetal heart checks. The monitor tape records the information.

### DISADVANTAGES

a) As we shall see later, the major risk to mother and child from electronic monitoring is Cesarean section and the ensuing risks of a surgical birth.

b) The accuracy of the external monitor is often questionable. Maintenance and calibration are uncertain. Also, for best results the woman usually must remain relatively immobile or the equipment must be checked after each change of position.

c) The mother cannot get out of bed, walk, sit in a rocking chair, or take a shower. Her lack of mobility may increase her discomfort, and it also constitutes a risk to the baby because of reduced maternal blood circulation. The side position, a favorite of laboring women, usually reduces the accuracy of the monitor. Most monitored patients are recumbent on their backs, a posture long known to interfere with maternal circulation (and therefore the infant's) as the heavy uterus rests on the vena cava, a major blood vessel. If the monitor shows a significant drop in the fetal heart rate, the woman is instructed to turn onto her side to aid the recovery of the baby's pulse. If the fetal heart rate remains low, Cesarean delivery will of course be considered. Thus, equipment malfunction has occasionally led to unnecessary surgery.

New monitors are being developed that a woman can walk around with during late pregnancy before labor even begins.

d) The presence of the monitor makes it hard for the woman to relax. Her level of stress may be increased. Some of the Lamaze comfort techniques involving light abdominal massage cannot be done because of the equipment.

e) The unfolding tape must be read continuously to be of any use. If it is ignored, it serves no purpose. If the tape is continually observed, direct auscultation (listening) to the baby by fetascope could as easily be done.

f) The unknown hazards of continuous ultrasound exposure during the hours of labor in addition to prenatal diagnostic ultrasound are not known. Experiments on animals focus attention on neurological effects and possible leukemia. Other possibilities are behavioral effects, genetic effects, and effects on the body's immune system. Studies are now being done, but the assumption of safety to date is based only on clinical impressions. Everyone agrees that ultrasound exposure is safer than X ray, but X rays themselves were once considered safe.

g) The monitor may contribute a dehumanizing aspect to the labor, as nurses and husband focus more on the beeping, flashing monitor endlessly disgorging its tape than on the woman herself. The husband may back off from his wife in deference to the machine. The atmosphere of tranquility may be replaced by a sense of urgency, tension, and even danger which, some hypothesize, may actually delay the progress of labor as the woman lies, nearly immobilized, with her hospital gown pushed up above the abdominal belt.

h) The constant attention to every heartbeat tends to emphasize the danger of labor to the baby, increasing the parents' worry.

i) The monitor permits the use of more Pitocin to speed labor than would normally be considered "safe." If the heart rate does not falter significantly, more Pitocin is added until its effect can be seen on the monitor. However, this may be far too much of the drug, since heart rate is not the sole indicator of fetal health. There is evidence showing that fetal distress may actually precede the drop in fetal heart rate by at least several minutes.

j) The monitor is hard for parents to refuse when it is presented for their baby's "safety" without the full story on the equipment's pros and cons. Patients are generally not informed about the known risks.

### INTERNAL ELECTRONIC FETAL HEART MONITOR

The internal monitor is more accurate, and when staff and patient become exasperated with the uncertain readings of the external monitor and the immobility it demands of the mother, an internal lead into the vagina is likely to be introduced. This development can produce a sense of disequilibrium for couples who had agreed that the external monitor only be used no more than necessary, possibly for a brief time if the nurse couldn't hear the baby adequately, or during an occasional contraction to see if the contractions affected the baby adversely.

The internal monitor has leads which are inserted into the vagina and attached to the scalp of the baby. If the membranes have not already ruptured spontaneously, they must be ruptured for the leads to be inserted. The monitor is usually attached soon after admission. If it is delayed a few hours until the membranes rupture spontaneously, as many parents request, the question arises, why attach it at all?

The internal monitor has many of the same advantages and disadvantages of the external monitor, except that the accuracy of the reading is improved and the woman's mobility may be increased. However, she still cannot get out of bed with the internal monitoring equipment that is now in use.

The monitor electrodes may be attached to the baby's scalp when the cervical dilation is 2 or 3 centimeters. An additional intrauterine catheter can also be introduced to gauge the relative strength of contractions as well as their frequency, although these readings are less accurate than those for the fetal heart rate. Nevertheless, if the catheter doesn't record contractions adjudged sufficiently strong, Pitocin may be given until they are. Then if the baby's heart rate falters after introducing Pitocin, the Pitocin may be turned off. If the heart rate does not recover, a Cesarean is done, the rationale being that the labor failed to progress and the monitor showed that the baby was in distress. There is also the small possibility of cord puncture with the intrauterine catheter.

The advantages, as previously stated, are the same as for the external monitor plus increased mobility and accuracy (if the equipment is in working order and properly calibrated).

### DISADVANTAGES

a) An amniotomy must be done before the electrodes can be placed under the skin of the fetal scalp. Therefore the length of the labor is automatically limited. Twenty-four hours or however long the hospital decides to "allow" labor to continue, may be long enough, but suppose the woman is not yet in real labor when the amniotomy is performed. An otherwise unnecessary Cesarean may occur, either because Pitocin is given as a result of using the monitor and the monitor measures potential fetal heart-rate problems from the Pitocin, or because the labor does not progress sufficiently fast after the amniotomy.

b) Infections do occur both for mother and infant. The official incidence is less than 1 percent, but some hospital staff report that the actual figure is higher. Conservative guesses are offered that the true infection rate is 10 percent, 20 percent, or more.

c) The electrodes may be accidentally implanted in an area other than the infant's scalp, such as the eyes, buttocks, or genitalia. Because most babies are head-down with the chin tucked under, these situations are rare, but they do occur. Obstetricians do not always know the position of the baby, even with ultrasound.

d) As with the external monitor, the stresses associated with being electronically monitored may act to slow labor, perhaps as a result of increased secretion of the chemical substance epinephrine by the mother's adrenal glands. Deep relaxation, so helpful in relieving pain, is more difficult to achieve, and chemical pain relief may be the solution.

e) All types of electronic monitoring, whether based on ultrasonography and electronics and whether external or internal, result in decreased options and some degree of dehumanization for the parents.

f) Monitoring is done based on the false assumption that every baby can be saved. If by remote chance the baby should die at this time, as shown by loss of fetal heartbeat, parents often do not want a still-born delivered by Cesarean section. They then must cope with two traumatic events: surgery and death of the infant.

g) Recent, well-controlled studies, including the widely heralded research by Dr. David Banta for the federal government's Office of Technology Assessment, have shown no benefit from monitoring normal women over periodic listening to the fetal heart with a stethoscope. Electronic monitoring was of benefit only to women in certain defined categories of risk, such as diabetes and prematurity.

The U. S. Government Health, Education and Welfare publication "Antenatal Diagnosis," 1979, states that the fetal heart-rate patterns on the monitor are not a high predictor of infant condition at birth as determined by the Apgar score. To diagnose fetal distress fetal heart information should be combined with the presence of meconium and results of a test on fetal scalp blood. This publication is the report of a conference sponsored by the National Institute of Child Health and Human Development. It also states: "In the low-risk population, the risk of infant death is so low that the low inherent risks of monitoring (0.6 lives per thousand) may outweigh the small increment of benefit." If monitoring were to be used for all of the three million U.S. births per year, 1,350 avoidable infant deaths would occur. Also, a study on fetal monitoring reported in the publication of the Harvard Medical Area *Focus* in December 1981 found striking differences among physicians in interpretation of the monitoring data, also a definite risk of unnecessary Cesarean section.

Informed parent input and consent are essential to help in making decisions about the use of technology. Parents can come to understand the issues every bit as well as the professionals, although the wishes of individual parents may differ. Some parents, knowing the possible problems of the monitor, will still want to use it.

On the other hand, obstetricians need parental support to bypass the monitor when labor is normal, the baby is not premature, the mother is not hypertensive or diabetic, there is no uterine bleeding, and hospital staff is available to check the fetal heart rate every few minutes and during a contraction.

Instead of monitors, frequent, direct listening to the fetal heart is recommended by many childbirth educators, with the suggestion that a device called a doptone be used selectively and intermittently. The doptone is placed on the woman's abdomen and uses brief exposure to ultrasound to listen to the baby's heart. The sounds are magnified to the point where they can be heard by anyone in the room, the rapid "lub-dups" being about twice the rate of the adult heart. The device is often used in the doctor's office during prenatal visits instead of the fetascope.

Monitoring equipment is not used in alternative birth centers. It is not used in most birth rooms since women with potentially problematic labors or deliveries aren't allowed to use the room anyway. In most hospitals, parents can refuse monitors with less argument than they can intravenous fluids.

## "WHY DO I NEED THE IV?"
## "WHY CAN'T I DRINK WATER?"

As with fetal heart monitoring, the assumption might be made that intravenous fluids, a routine, apparently harmless procedure, would be used only when medically indicated for the patient's own good. It could even be assumed that since the IV is a medical procedure, decisions about its use are best made by hospital personnel. For several years, the vehemence of the hospital's insistence on an intravenous for virtually every woman in labor has sparked consumer health groups to explore this apparently innocuous procedure.

Like the monitor, an IV has become an almost routine hospital admission procedure, reimbursable by health insurance. Unlike the monitor, it as yet shows little sign of being phased out, except in alternative birth centers and birth rooms, and in certain hospitals.

Usually, the IV remains in place throughout labor and for an hour or two afterward, the needle in a vein in the wrist or the back of the hand. Some women have it taped to a board on their forearms to help keep the needle in its proper place as it drips continuously from the bottle suspended from a bedside pole.

The obvious question, "Why is it so difficult to avoid the IV if it's not needed?" parallels the question, "Why is it so hard to get truly natural childbirth?" There are factors involved beyond the patient's physiological need for adequate water.

The ratios of cost, benefit, and risk of using IVs on all maternity patients have not been studied. Risks are unseen or discounted. How could there possibly be any harm in putting water and sugar into anyone at any time for that matter? Some of the patients are bound to get dehydrated, especially if labor lasts a long while and no food or drink is allowed. So it is seen as a preventive measure suitable for all.

The reasons given for ordering an IV are not exactly the same as the real reasons, but medical practitioners are exposed to these rationales so often that they may not question them. The reasons given include:

a) "The IV gives nutrition."

The dextrose or glucose and water in no way replaces a meal. There are no vitamins, no minerals, no protein in an IV. It does not give remotely the nutrition or the feeling of well-being that a glass of orange juice or milk might provide. Also, prolonged use of an IV alone can alter the electrolyte balance in the body. The assumption that IVs provide nutrition has allowed many hospital patients to receive insufficient nourishment over many hours. In fact, a study of surgical patients showed that many experienced slowed postoperative recovery because of an insufficient supply of protein.

b) "Digestion stops during labor."

No study indicates that this is true. During late first stage, the transition and second stage, digestion may be slowed, and throughout labor, fear, pain, and exposure to a strange environment may inhibit feelings of hunger. Drugged women, of course, may be in no condition to eat or drink, but many undrugged women report that their hunger during labor reached the point of being uncomfortable. Many couples now bring fluids or ice chips to the hospital, even if they are not "allowed" to, hoping that a trusted nurse or obstetrician will look the other way.

c) "The IV doesn't hurt."

True, but one's hand may get a bit puffy, and over a period of hours there may be some discomfort. Also, it can be a nuisance to keep track of so that it doesn't get hooked on the bed or accidentally yanked out.

d) "She can still walk."

Yes, as long as the husband or a friend walks beside her holding the stand and the bottle (and assuming that no monitor is in place).

**e)** "She shouldn't have anything by mouth. She might vomit and aspirate it."

Part of the intimidating effect of the IV is the message it delivers that henceforth the woman can have nothing orally, no matter how dry her mouth is or how long the labor. (The IV does not remedy the "cotton mouth" resulting from several hours of labor breathing.) Thus, the IV adds the fear of choking to the traditional fears about pain.

Women may experience a transitory nausea, or may even vomit, during transition, although this is uncommon. It may result from a long period of having an empty stomach, or from a huge meal eaten just prior to labor, or for no apparent reason at all. This nausea can be handled as well in labor as at other times in life and does not usually result from small amounts of food. In fact, prolonged fasting may actually increase nausea.

Most hospitals still allow ice chips. Some now offer juices. A few do not permit even ice chips, substituting an antacid substance such as Maalox. The rationale: "Better she should inhale an alkaline substance than the acids of her stomach. She could get lung damage from the acid." Some obstetricians in these hospitals order ice chips anyway and tell their patients to throw the Maalox away.

(If vomit is somehow inhaled, the pH must be lower than 2.5, on a total pH scale of 0–14, 7 being neutral, to injure lung tissue and thereby produce a pneumonic condition.)

In many birth rooms and in all alternative birth centers, where there is no reason for an IV, women may eat and drink whatever they wish (although they often have to bring their own food).

**f)** "She might hemorrhage and we couldn't find a vein, especially if she went into shock."

Life-saving skills are highly valued. They form the bedrock of the trust and power that society gives to the medical profession. The preceding statement, if nothing else, can evoke fear in parents for whom the fear of the hemorrhage follows a close third to the fear of pain and fear of a birth defect. It causes fear in obstetricians also if the record shows that the standard IV was not in place prior to the bleeding. Malpractice possibilities, of course, have an impact on medical treatment and its costs. An IV can solve a problem for a few patients, and therefore it is seen as necessary for everyone. Because the procedure is a standard one accepted by the profession, physicians feel safer if they use IVs in the same way they still often feel safer if they use a monitor.

Hemorrhaging can be life-threatening, immediately and visibly so. However, it is not associated with normal birth. A woman is more likely to hemorrhage if she is undernourished or malnourished. Hemorrhage is also more likely with the use of spinal, epidural, or gas anesthesia. It is associated with the rare condition of the placenta detaching during labor, as with placenta previa or placenta abruptio, as described in Chapter One, under "Possible Medical Problems." In these cases, bleeding during labor is a signal that a Cesarean may have to be done quickly, and an IV is needed.

However, most serious hemorrhages occur after birth, not during labor. The woman does not go into shock before a vein can be found to insert fluid or blood. Usually the uterus is held tightly by the obstetrician. An IV may be inserted at this time if needed. Moreover, a device may be inserted during labor to "keep a vein open," a constant refrain of hospital staff. No IV need be attached to it until when and if an IV is necessary.

After birth, an IV Pitocin may routinely be given to contract the uterus and prevent further bleeding, just as earlier the IV Pitocin may have been used to induce or speed the labor. The alternative is to check to see whether the uterus has already contracted and to station a recovery-room nurse responsible for checking newly delivered women, especially those who have had regional (spinal, epidural, or saddle block) anesthesia. Finally, Pitocin can also be given by needle. Even if the drug is indicated in a particular case, there's no need to introduce it intravenously.

The above are the ostensible reasons for giving intravenous fluids. More central are the following reasons, which are less accessible to both health professionals and parents.

a) Many physicians will tell you that they feel liable if an IV is not in place. It will be needed eventually if the labor is long and the woman isn't allowed anything to eat or drink, or if regional anesthesia—spinal, saddle block, or epidural—is to be used. They feel especially liable if the IV is not in place after birth for the introduction of Pitocin to "shrink the uterus," because they are not present after the birth, not even for five minutes in almost every instance. After suturing the episiotomy and writing a note on the chart, the obstetrician is ordinarily gone. Obstetricians depend on the nurse to check the patient's uterus and the sanitary pad used to catch the flow. He needs the IV for his protection. Only the patient can refuse it.

b) Every aspect of hospital life supports the use of the IV. It is seen as preventive. It is reimbursable by insurance companies. It is an established medical procedure. Colleagues do it. The Anesthesiology Department, usually not highly visible and with little say in decisions about birth, may extend two very visible regulations: One allows nothing by mouth after hospital admission, and the second stipulates that every woman have an IV.

c) The expediency of the routine IV during and after the birth, which frees the physician from having to worry about every patient, has an appeal to the obstetrician. He spends his day on the run, involved in many separate interactions. The statement is often made, "Nothing is routine in medicine," when patients ask if monitors, episiotomies, or IVs are routine. The fact is that there *are* medical routines that are beginning to be deeply questioned.

d) Obstetricians do not wish to question the IV and nothing-by-mouth requirements of the anesthesiologists. This is not their territory, although they are responsible for the birth. If pressed, they may write an order for ice chips or refrain from ordering an IV, however. The obstetricians need not only patients, but also a place to bring them. They do not care to antagonize any other segment of the hospital. Only parents can interrupt the routine use of the IV for childbirth.

e) The legal system makes it difficult for patients to take ultimate responsibility for the outcome of their medical care. They cannot waive their right to sue. They can refuse procedures, but if the patient's judgment proves faulty, the physician or hospital or both may still be legally liable. The medical experts are presumed to know best, especially if the procedure is a routine one.

f) Physicians feel threatened by their patient's involvement in a strictly medical procedure. They fail to see the reason for the parents' objection to an IV, other than an irrational fear of a needle that could conceivably save the mother's life. It was hard for physicians to accept patients' refusal of drugs, but the general knowledge that drugs can be dangerous, and the fact that patients can sue for drugs given that they have refused, makes the refusal of pain medications easier than refusing the apparently innocuous IV.

## Why Do Some Parents Object to the Routine Use of Intravenous Fluids?

**a)** The length of time allowed for labor is shortened, although this result is more subtle than in the case of the internal fetal heart monitor where someone decides, somewhat arbitrarily, how long the membrane can be ruptured with the electrodes in the fetal scalp before a Cesarean is done. As bottles of IV fluid are emptied, a sense of urgency tends to prevail. How long can one lie on a bed, nothing-by-mouth, relatively immobile, with the IV dripping its fluid? The tendency toward immobility may affect the fetal heart rate. An intermittent labor over two or three days may present no significant problem if the woman is up and about while continuing to carry on light activity, but this pattern cannot be followed with IV, which usually remains in place until after delivery. If she wishes to walk, someone must carry the pole and IV bottle for her.

**b)** Once an IV is in place, the temptation to speed labor by adding Pitocin becomes almost irresistible for both staff and parents.

**c)** The bladder, which at term can hold only a few teaspoons or less of urine, fills during labor whether or not food and drink are offered and whether or not an IV is used, but the IV fills the bladder faster. If the bladder isn't emptied, labor progress may be inhibited and the pain of contractions increased. It is usually no one's responsibility other than the husband's to get the woman up to the bathroom on a regular basis. The woman may not be "allowed" to walk because her membrane has ruptured or been broken even if the baby's head is engaged and there is no possibility of umbilical cord compression. The order may not be a physician's order or a written policy from any part of the hospital; but if a nurse says no bathroom privileges, this directive usually prevails. So, amidst wires and tubes, the woman may have to balance on a bedpan.

Moreover, the full bladder's effect of delaying labor and increasing pain may be attacked by Pitocin and pain medication, and perhaps with epidural anesthesia and a forceps delivery.

d) No study indicates the need for a routine IV. No study supports the nothing-by-mouth ritual unless gas, instead of spinal or epidural, anesthesia is used in the event of a Cesarean. No standards for the use of an IV have been developed to take advantage of its very real benefits in defined situations.

e) The IV highlights the power of the institution over the parents. The woman, tethered to her bottle, along with other instrumentation, appears more like a captive or a very sick patient than a woman hiring professional services for a normal birth.

f) No study indicates that food cannot be digested during labor, except possibly during very active labor. The common statement, "It just sits like a lump in her stomach," has no known basis in fact, other than the common knowledge that anxiety can inhibit digestion.

g) The use of the IV allows the continuation of the "nothing-by-mouth" requirement, yet doesn't significantly relieve "cotton mouth," a major discomfort of labor. For some the IV is a reason for having a home birth. Others eat and drink before coming to the hospital. One woman told me:

> "If I'd had a drink at the bubbler before we signed in, it would have been okay. Because we had already been admitted, the nurse literally grabbed me away from the drinking fountain. Thirst was the most uncomfortable part of my labor."

Marathon runners, whose muscles are obviously working, contracting to the maximum, commonly drink copiously during their run. No one expects them to have fluids introduced by vein.

h) Most parents haven't a clue that the IV might lead to a full bladder, a tendency toward immobility, or any of the other procedures such as the administering of Pitocin or an epidural, all of which can add to the possibility of a Cesarean. The route is indirect, but those who analyze labor in its entirety and question the reasons for the currently high Cesarean rate must conclude that even the innocuous-appearing IV is implicated.

i) Research at Georgetown University concludes that the sugar in the IV causes the mother's pancreas to secrete extra insulin, resulting in hypoglycemia in the newborn which, ironically, is treated by giving the baby sugar water.

On the other hand, an IV is indicated in the case of spinal or epidural anesthesia, a Cesarean section, a uterus that does not contract well after birth, or an inability to give the mother fluids in any other way.

An IV will be useful if labor is long, especially if the woman arrived at the hospital on an empty stomach. The IV is not often a major physical discomfort during labor. The objection is rather that a useful and life-saving procedure has become a routine "preventive" measure that may even prevent spontaneous birth, since the possible problems from routine use may not be addressed. The labyrinthian route to possible induced labor, pain, fetal distress, regional anesthesia, and Cesarean is indirect and not measurable. Ironically, the immobility encouraged by IVs and monitors can promote slowing of the fetal heart, the very risk most interventions are designed to combat. Couples who decide to have a baby and make the foray into the unknown territories of childbirth and medicine should be aware that the outcome of the birth is not dependent solely on anatomy and physiology.

## PITOCIN

Since Pitocin affects many aspects of labor and delivery, it has already been mentioned in relation to the induction of labor, anesthesia, and intravenous fluids. A controversial, yet sometimes useful drug, it requires more complete discussion here.

One of more than a dozen hormones secreted by the pituitary gland, oxytocin is involved in the normal beginning of labor and in the Braxton Hicks contractions prior to labor. During sexual activity, oxytocin is involved in orgasm and ejaculation. During breast-feeding it initiates the let-down reflex which brings milk from the milk-producing glands down where the baby can get it.

(See "The Breast and Breast-feeding" in Chapter Six.) Synthetic oxytocin is marketed most frequently under the name Pitocin, or Syntocinon.

The *Physicians' Desk Reference* (or *PDR*), a volume on every practicing physician's desk, describes Pitocin as a "substance with antidiuretic properties affecting uterine motility." It is suitable for medically required (as opposed to elective) induction of labor such as preeclampsia, prematurely ruptured membranes, and to reinforce labor in selected cases of uterine inertia.

Contraindications, according to the *PDR,* are significant CPD (when the fetal head is too large for the pelvis) and when the fetal position makes the baby undeliverable (as in a transverse position). Patients with obstetrical emergencies where the benefit-to-risk ratio for mother or fetus favors surgical intervention should not receive Pitocin. For example, if there is fetal distress early in labor, a Cesarean would be indicated, not Pitocin to speed labor. Other contraindications are prolonged use for uterine inertia when the uterus is not contracting effectively, or severe toxemia, or for hypertonic uterine patterns, meaning that the uterine muscle tone is more than adequate, even irritable. Hypersensitivity to the drug is a contraindication, as is cord presentation (when the cord is seen before the birth of the baby).

The *PDR* states that Pitocin, when given for induction or stimulation of labor, must be administered only by the intravenous route (for controlled administration as opposed to giving a "shot") with adequate medical supervision in a hospital. Patients must be under continuous observation by trained personnel. A physician qualified to manage any complications should be immediately available.

The *PDR* states that maternal deaths due to hypertensive episodes and rupture of the uterus, and fetal deaths due to various causes have been reported as a result of use of Pitocin for induction or augmentation of the first and second stages of labor.

Oxytocin has been shown to have an antidiuretic effect. Attention should be given to the possibility of water intoxication, a condition in which excess water in the tissues leads to a serious biochemical imbalance, particularly when the oxytoxic substance is administered continually by infusion and the patient is receiving fluids by mouth.

The *PDR* reports adverse reactions such as slowed fetal heart rate, postpartum hemorrhage, pelvic bruises, and irregular maternal heartbeat. Excess dosage or hypersensitivity to the drug may result in uterine spasm, tetanic contraction (a strong, sustained contraction that does not subside in a minute), or rupture.

Side effects of Pitocin are "nausea, vomiting, and possibility of increased blood loss. Severe water intoxication with slow infusion over a 24-hour period has been reported to result in maternal death."

Pitocin, as has been stated, is used in many hospitals almost routinely (in 70–80 percent of women) to induce or augment labor, and is used routinely (in almost 100 percent of women) after birth to contract the uterus and prevent postpartum bleeding. It is ironic that Pitocin, used to control postpartum bleeding, is associated with increased postpartum bleeding when used during labor.

Although not reported by the *PDR,* Pitocin stimulation has also been associated with respiratory problems of the newborn and the relatively common newborn jaundice (see Chapter Five), as well as increased pain for the mother.

Pitocin is generally used in cases of uterine dystocia, or "lazy" uterus. The notation on the medical record may be "failure to progress." However, there is no real agreement on what constitutes sufficient labor progress, despite the expected, but often unrealistic, dilation of 1 centimeter per hour discussed earlier. Labors differ. If some are faster than average, it follows that some must be slower. The earlier the couple goes to the hospital, especially because labor often starts with infrequent and irregular contractions, the more likely the label "failure to progress" is applied.

Prepared couples, if the labor is described as "doing nothing" or "going nowhere" or who have long-ruptured membranes, usually prefer to use physiological methods to encourage labor first. These methods include relaxation, changing position, taking a walk or a warm shower, or perhaps even going home. Long, slow labors are difficult to manage in a hospital setting.

Patients are no longer ordinarily admitted to private rooms but are admitted directly to labor and delivery. In traditional settings there are no lawn chairs, lounges, or movies. Physicians desire a defined, predictable end to the labor for planning purposes. Physicians desire a healthy outcome reasonably soon. An unpublished study of one large institution showed that significantly more babies were born between 9 A.M. and 5 P.M. Clearly, this is the result of intervention.

Besides being used to speed labor, Pitocin may be used to effect stronger, more frequent contractions. It may be used to save the mother from a possible Cesarean because of a previous amniotomy or spontaneous membrane rupture. Conversely, the use of Pitocin may result in a Cesarean if it puts the baby under stress. In any case, the use of Pitocin automatically places the woman in a high-risk category whether or not she was high risk before the drug was given.

## A FINAL WORD ON OBSTETRICAL INTERVENTIONS DURING LABOR

The technology can be life-saving. This statement is made frequently, and it is true. Needed in certain circumstances are ways to start labor, to give fluids to incapacitated women, to give blood, to monitor the baby, and to remove the baby surgically.

However when they are used without adequate standards or cause, normal labors may be altered in ways that require further intervention. Risks, including that of surgery, are increased subtly. Amidst the web of labor procedures this may not be clearly perceived by the hospital staff, who are caught up with the immediacy of daily tasks and responsibilities. Therefore, leadership in this area can often best come from outside the institution. Inside the hospital, there is no one (with the possible exception of midwives, and their professional position is still in many instances precarious) with the responsibility of overseeing a patient's total situation and minimizing unnecessary risks. However, individual couples, if they have the knowledge, can alter this pattern.

# Chapter Five

# DELIVERY PROCEDURES

The day of birth is a special time for woman, man, baby, and everyone else who attends the momentous event. What occurs at delivery will depend partly on what has happened during labor. It will depend also on prior planning on the part of the parents.

## PLACE OF DELIVERY

### Delivery Room

The place of delivery will depend on the facilities available and on whether or not a normal delivery is anticipated. A few couples will select an alternative birth center or their own home. These new options will be discussed in Chapter Nine.

As the tempo of labor picks up at transition, so does the activity of the nurses. During labor, the nurses check the mother's blood pressure and the fetal heart, and monitor the contractions and the degree of cervical dilation. If IVs and Pitocin, or other medications are used, nurses will be involved, here, too. If a monitor is used, nurses will keep an eye on it. When delivery is imminent, the obstetrician must be called by a nurse. When the moment of birth is only minutes away, with the baby's head perhaps already showing, the woman may be moved to the delivery room. Her husband exchanges his own clothes for hospital garb like that of the obstetrician. (The sooner the father-to-be changes clothes, the less likely is he to have to leave his wife for this purpose at a critical time when she needs coaching for every contraction.) At the delivery room door he may be handed paper shoes, a paper hat, and a mask for his nose and mouth.

An atmosphere of crisis typically prevails in late labor as nurses decide when to call the doctor, move the mother, adjust the table, drape her legs, unwrap instruments for the episiotomy, set up the IV for postpartum use if it wasn't administered during labor, get the anesthesiologist, and so on and so forth. The atmosphere appears closer to chaos than calm.

Most delivery rooms still have the traditional surgical table onto which the mother climbs, or is rolled onto, from the labor bed—which is then wheeled back into the hall outside the delivery room. (She may take the pillows from the bed before it is removed.) This room is an operating room and contains a lot of equipment, bottles, tubes, and stainless steel, most of which will not be used. Nevertheless, it may appear intimidating at first.

## Birth Room

Most parents who know about birth rooms prefer them to delivery rooms. An obstetrician, Philip Summer of Connecticut, pioneered in the early 1970s the then-novel idea of allowing parents to deliver in the same room they have labored in. The purpose is to avoid disturbing them when labor is active and they prefer to concentrate on the impending birth.

If a midwife is delivering, she will already be there. If a physician is attending, he or she must be called, but in the birth room the obstetrician is less likely to be gowned and scrubbed. He will probably wear sterile gloves, however. The husband seldom changes clothes or is masked. The mother's knees and abdomen are not draped. There may be a birth chair, instead of a birth bed. If desired, stirrups can be screwed onto the birth-room bed, but they seldom are. The physician leans over the bed, sits on the end of it, or even kneels on the floor to deliver the baby. The woman may have a pocket mirror to help her see the birth, or she may be raised enough on her knees or elbows to see for herself. This helps her decide, with others in the room, whether there is need to push and with how much force. There is an atmosphere of excitement over the imminent arrival of the baby. If, at any time, there is need for delivery-room equipment, it can be made available, or the mother can go to the delivery room. Hospitals that do not yet have a birth room may permit delivery in one of the labor rooms.

Anesthesia, other than local, is not used in birth rooms. Often there is no episiotomy, no IV. There will not be a monitor, because if the mother is high risk, she will not be in the birth room in the first place. After delivery, the baby stays in the room for a time, depending on the wishes of the parents or the staff's need for the room.

## POSITION FOR DELIVERY

Prospective parents usually discuss the position for delivery with their obstetrician when planning the birth. More commonly now the mother may deliver in the position of her choice, unless a general anesthetic is required.

### Lithotomy

Informed women usually wish to avoid this traditional hospital birth position for delivery. In this position, the woman lies on her back with her knees separated and her legs supported in stirrups or in leg supports resembling one half of an orthopedic leg cast. Her shoulders can be raised with a couple of pillows. Some women use the stirrups to push against and therefore find the position workable, especially if the supports are adjusted as low as possible to be in line with her body.

The lithotomy position allows the physician access to the vagina with forceps. It is also required before epidural or spinal anesthesia is administered. And after a spinal, the woman will remain flat to minimize the possibility of a spinal headache.

The lithotomy position also facilitates the episiotomy incision and may, in fact, require it because of the stretch it places on the perineum, the area between the anus and the vagina. To sum up, the lithotomy position usually requires an episiotomy, and an episiotomy usually requires the lithotomy position.

### Semi-sitting

In this position, the woman's back is curved, with her head and shoulders raised and a pillow beneath each knee. Her legs are apart, but not so wide that there is excessive stretch on the pelvic tissues.

## Side Position

In this position, the woman lies on her side with her husband helping to support the top leg. This position minimizes stretch on the perineum. Also, it makes it easy for her husband to apply back pressure if her back is sore. This position aids circulation to the placenta, especially if the mother lies on her left side.

## All-fours Position

For some women, this may be the only comfortable position for labor and delivery. The mother may fold her arms and rest them on two or three pillows, or spread her knees and squat down with her shoulders higher than her hips.

## Birth Chairs

These chairs, which resemble in some ways Colonial birthing stools, have an area of the seat cut out to allow delivery.

## Squatting

Birth may be hastened by squatting with the feet twelve to eighteen inches apart and with the heels flat on the floor and the pelvic floor relaxed. The baby is brought down close to the surface of the body when squatting. The woman requires support in this position, especially if she is on a bed, and it cannot usually be maintained for many minutes at a time. During labor some women squat temporarily on the floor with their backs supported by the wall of the room.

The position for delivery is important. As long ago as 1964, a study showed that the semi-squatting position minimized pain and shortened the second stage of labor. In the case of a large baby or a posterior baby, the position is especially important.

One woman told me:

"For my first baby with epidural anesthesia I just couldn't push the baby down. It was partly the anesthesia, I know, and the Pitocin they used slowed the baby's heart rate from 140 down to close to a 100. I know the baby's heart rate dips slightly during a contraction anyhow, but the Pitocin really affected it. I ended up with a Cesarean. Later, when I thought about it I remembered that at the beginning of the second stage before the epidural, it had felt good to push when I was sitting on the john, as though I was making progress. Then back in bed flat on my back again it hurt to push and I couldn't seem to make any headway. For my second baby I got into a squatting position, not the semi-sitting position even, and I had no trouble at all pushing her out. She was a bigger baby, too."

# EPISIOTOMY

This minor but controversial surgical procedure is an incision to enlarge the vaginal opening. It is interrelated with other birth procedures such as anesthesia and position for birth.

The cut is made with scissors. The blade is placed in the vagina, and several snips are made. The direction may be down (median) toward the rectum and even occasionally through the rectum. Some incisions will tear through the rectum if the mother pushes hard, especially in the lithotomy position.

The incision may instead be made diagonally out to the side (mediolateral), in which case the cut may be extended farther than the median episiotomy. This type causes more pain in healing, and some obstetricians say more infections result from this mediolateral incision.

The incision may be a first-degree cut, which includes only the perineal skin and vaginal mucous membrane. Or it may be a second-degree incision, including as well the perineal muscles around the vagina, or a third-degree cut, involving skin, mucous membrane, perineal muscle, and anal sphincter.

The episiotomy is often preceded by a splash of chilly, brown antiseptic solution. The unexpected cold splash may cause a tightening of the pelvic-floor muscles just when they need to be released for birth.

Tears if they should occur do not usually involve muscle. Most obstetricians do the second-degree incision, which may be about two inches long. Some obstetricians tend to make longer ones, and there is little correlation between the physiologic situation and the procedure used.

If a woman requests that there be no episiotomy, the answer may be, "I only do them when they are necessary." In practice, somehow, they always seem to be necessary—except when she delivers the baby's head before the procedure can be done. Even with the head fully crowned, an incision may be made. What makes the procedure "necessary" is not defined. Most obstetricians are still trained to believe that every woman needs one. Consequently, they have no criteria for knowing when they need not be done. Not all women object to a small tear which can be stitched and is not felt anyway.

The fundamental reason for the episiotomy was originally the anesthetized birth requiring forceps to extract the baby. To introduce forceps the episiotomy was required. Conversely the use of forceps requires anesthesia.

Many obstetricians are still trained to deliver with routine episiotomy, and it does speed delivery by a couple of minutes. More physicians and parents are beginning to question them, especially as they are not done routinely by nurse-midwives or lay midwives (see Chapter Eight).

Although these hypotheses have not been substantiated by research, the rationale for routine episiotomies goes as follows:

a) Episiotomies are supposed to prevent the pounding of the baby's head against the perineum which "could cause brain damage." The use of outlet forceps for the last contraction is said to be safer. This reasoning, however, assumes that all women are tense and frightened, holding their legs together and tightly clenching their pelvic-floor muscles.

b) A permanently enlarged vagina may supposedly result if no episiotomy is done, and it is feared that subsequent sexual enjoyment—especially that of the husband—will be diminished, a theory unproven by science. This also assumes a non-prepared woman with no control of her own musculature who never does Kegel exercises (which should be done by everyone, man or woman, throughout life). It assumes that an episiotomy will prevent the so-called enlarged vagina, but no study shows this.

c) A jagged tear, which could result from not having an episiotomy, is said to be harder to repair than a straight incision. If the incision or the tear were very large, this might be true, but the woman will not know the difference if sufficient time and care are taken for the repair. Moreover, a tear is unlikely in the case of a controlled delivery with gentle, steady pushing.

d) Some physicians say, "Her pelvic organs may fall out later in life," meaning that the bladder or rectum protrude into the vaginal space. If there should be need to repair or reposition pelvic organs, it is only a minor surgical procedure. At times this surgery has been required, but these women were delivered mostly under general anesthesia with forceps. They were never taught how to push during labor or about Kegel exercises to strengthen the pelvic floor. Most of these women, moreover, had episiotomies for birth.

In impoverished countries where malnutrition is prevalent, prolapse, in which the uterus actually dropped out of the body, has been observed both among women who have never borne children at all and among women who have borne many children under poor conditions. No study shows that this problem has any relationship to the practice of episiotomy.

e) Episiotomy is claimed to shorten the second stage of labor by one to five minutes. Yes, it does, mostly because it allows the introduction of forceps, but also because it widens the birth canal and thus allows the baby to be pushed out faster. The benefits of routinely shortening labor in this way are questionable.

The routine episiotomy has affected childbirth procedures beyond the surgery itself and the postpartum recovery. For years it was responsible for the handcuffing of both anesthetized and awake women to delivery tables so that they would not touch the birth area or the baby. Legs were restrained to prevent her from struggling against the surgery, although anesthesia effectively did this.

The episiotomy was also responsible for the use of sterile drapes for all births. These were, and still are in many cases, placed over the woman's abdomen and knees, thereby making it impossible for her to see the lower part of her body and to assume the appropriate body positions for pushing. The drapes were used so that the obstetrician would not disturb the sterile field if he touched her leg or abdomen with his sterile glove and so that he could place sterile suturing materials on her abdomen. Even today, women who touch the sterile sheets may be reprimanded severely without explanation as well as without cause. Some women, wishing to view birth unobstructed, or even to catch their own babies instead of simply being a surgical patient, request that no drapes be used on the legs or abdomen.

Episiotomies also justified the use of masks in the delivery room (for everyone except the mother), because surgery was being performed. However, the episiotomy may introduce bacteria into the vagina, and both the incision and the placental site are vulnerable to infection in this way.

Episiotomies were used to justify the shaving of the pubic area long after it was recognized that that practice bore no relationship to childbed fever. The shaving may not even be necessary in the case of an episiotomy unless there is hair that may be sewn into the stitches, but shaving is associated with an expected episiotomy.

Recovery from episiotomy adds days to a woman's hospital stay, painful days during which she must learn "peri care" to keep the stitches clean. She learns about sprays, warm sitz baths, donuts to sit on, and ice to relieve swelling and pain. Her ability to care for her infant can be affected. It is hard to sit, hard to walk, hard to go to the bathroom. Breast-feeding starts with the handicap of a sore bottom along with possibly sore nipples. This pain, often lasting without letup over several days, can be as distressing as labor pain, or even more so. No medications really help. Episiotomy pain tends to increase fears about pain in childbirth among women who are anesthetized for birth. "I'm sure glad I took the epidural. I could barely walk for days after I had my baby," these women say.

Careful suturing in the reconstruction of the vagina with painstaking matching of tissues and the application of ice soon after the surgery can minimize the pain.

A woman's sex life is affected by an episiotomy. Numbness from the severed nerves is likely to last for an indeterminate length of time and may delay the desire for resumption of sexual intercourse. Early attempts at intercourse after an episiotomy may cause pain, and lubrication with K-Y jelly may be required. Sometimes the woman is "stitched too tight," and the tissue may need to be stretched, in which case the obstetrician may be consulted. Eventually the problems recede, but they appear at a time when a woman may not relish coping with a sore bottom.

## Need for Episiotomy

When is an episiotomy genuinely required? Sometimes the baby descends so fast that there is no time for the gradual stretching of the tissues (although fast births can occur with no tearing). Sometimes the tissues begin to pale as they are tightly stretched, turning from deep pink to a whitish color. Sometimes when prodded gently they appear tight without the pliability to be moved over the baby's head. In such a case, the woman might only need to change her position. However, sometimes she is unable to stop pushing to allow the tissues to stretch gradually or she continues to push throughout delivery instead of gently for a few seconds at a time. Sometimes she has not been taught how to push properly or is not being coached. Sometimes she needs an episiotomy because tissues will not stretch or a medical problem requires a forceps delivery.

A tear cannot always be predicted. If there is a tear, it can be repaired, whether it is jagged or straight. In fact, a tear may be no more extensive than the routine episiotomy, which involves cutting muscle. A previous episiotomy, or more than one, does not require that an episiotomy be done for subsequent babies. The tissue of the incision has lost its elasticity, but it is strong tissue and the remainder of the sphincter tissues can expand adequately.

Some obstetricians when checking for tears not only examine the external tissues, but also reach in and pull down the cervix to check for lacerations. Most obstetricians feel that this is not desirable and do not do this. When the episiotomy has been repaired the obstetrician leaves.

There is no research on problems associated with episiotomy. The U. S. Government Office of Technology Assessment has begun a literature search. Most information is on types of incisions or suturing materials only. No long-term follow up has been published.

In a pamphlet published by the National Childbirth Trust in England, Sheila Kitzinger has published a summary of the reports of over a thousand women. It documents the known problems. She states also that episiotomy does not avoid tears or improve the condition of the perineum. She reports further that women have used alcohol prior to intercourse during the months after childbirth to cope with painful intercourse. Twenty-two percent reported painful intercourse three months after delivery. In English hospitals, midwives do deliveries including episiotomies. The requirement that an obstetrician do the subsequent suturing results for many women in a wait of several hours with an unstitched incision.

## Forceps

Forceps have been discussed in connection both with anesthetized birth and as being the original reason for the episiotomy.

The federal government is involved with the use of forceps (and vacuum extractors used often in other countries in preference to forceps) through its responsibility for regulating devices, funding research, and evaluating medical care. In 1976, the Medical Device Amendment made the FDA responsible for ensuring that medical devices are safe and effective, and forceps come under this law. Standards, however, regulate materials used rather than the occasions of their use. The American College of Obstetrics and Gynecology has yet to make a statement on standards for use of forceps. ACOG has commented, however, that, in its opinion, no increased problems result from the use of low forceps and that they offer advantages.

There is no easy way to study whether forceps are used correctly. Correlation between forceps and brain damage is difficult to assess, as are studies showing any possible advantages. The question is, Are they needed, and why?

High-forceps deliveries (before the head is engaged in the pelvis) are rarely if ever used at present. A Cesarean would be done instead. Mid-forceps delivery, where the head is engaged in the pelvis but not visible, is not common either. A Cesarean will be done if other efforts to bring down the baby are ineffective. In a low-forceps delivery, the head is visible and distends the vaginal opening.

Forceps come in many different types, but all consist of two long-handled spoon-shaped blades inserted separately along the sides of the baby's head. They are then locked together, and the baby's head is pulled gently through the vaginal opening.

Forceps were the original tool of obstetricians, one not available to midwives. Their almost magical ability to extract stuck infants was, and is, respected.

## Perineal Support and Massage
### An Alternative to Episiotomy

Support of birth-area tissues was a technique in use long before twentieth-century obstetrics evolved. However, it has now become a "new" technique, an alternative to routine episiotomy. Some obstetricians are beginning to add this technique, which consists simply of supporting the perineum (the area between the vagina and the anus) as the baby passes through, to their repertoire, having acquired it from midwives. The doctor supports the perineal area with his hand as the baby's head emerges, as if he were guiding a sweater over the baby's head. The baby is not held back; nor is the perineum pulled. Rather, the tissues are gently pressed or massaged away from the baby's head on all sides of the vagina, especially just below it. Warm, wet compresses may be used, the pressure and the warmth both helping to relax the pelvic-floor muscles and decrease the chance of a tear. Warm oil, especially vitamin E oil, is sometimes massaged into the perineum for lubrication and to aid elasticity. A couple of fingers gently pressing into the lower part of the vagina can identify tension in this area and help to relieve it. This pressure can also help the woman to focus the direction of her pushing.

Husbands may provide the support with warm, wet towels on the perineum. Nurses may help. The woman, if undraped and raised up enough to use her own hands, may herself support the tissues with her hands, and this may help her to know when to stop pushing. Photographs of this method of birth often show many hands providing an enveloping kind of support for her shoulders, her knees, and the bulging, stretching perineum.

## PARENT OPTIONS AT DELIVERY

The impact on parents of being the first to touch their own baby can be great, and this possibility is beginning to become a reality in hospital birth as well as in home birth and other options for birth. When the baby's head is about to crown, the woman may be asked if she would like to touch her baby. This can also help guide the direction of her expulsive efforts toward the vagina, not the rectum. The feeling of the warm, wet head lets her know her baby is almost born. The husband may also touch the baby at this time.

Sometimes after the baby's head and shoulders are out, the mother may be given the opportunity to "catch" her own baby.

"I saw the baby between my legs," one mother recalls. "I reached down to pick him up and realized the rest of him was still inside!" Obstetricians have been known to step aside for fathers to catch their babies.

As a symbolic gesture, the husband is often the one to cut the cord after it has been clamped. There is no reason the father instead of the obstetrician cannot perform this simple act. The new parents may feel an unexpected surge of emotion when birth is made less clinical, and find tears are running down their cheeks.

## CORD-CLAMPING

It is still possible that the traditional sequence of events at birth may occur. The emergence of the baby, the placing of the two cord clamps, the cutting of the cord with scissors, the handing of the baby to the nurse who places him or her in a box or infant warmer can all occur, almost with one motion, within seconds of birth. The woman on the table can't see the baby. The new father wonders if he is allowed to walk to the box in the corner to view the baby or must remain at his wife's head.

A benefit of delayed cord-cutting is that the baby's oxygen supply is not suddenly cut off, thus requiring that the baby take a first breath within seconds after birth. An additional benefit is that, for reasons not known, it seems to aid the placenta in separating from the uterus more quickly.

Most parents and professionals now believe that the cord should not be clamped immediately. The origin of rapid clamping may have been one of expediency. It was also related to the ether medications given the mother, which acted to depress the newborn's breathing. The desire was to minimize the amount reaching the baby through the placenta and cord.

If the cord is not clamped and cut immediately, the baby will of necessity remain with the parents on the birth bed. The baby will be placed on the mother's abdomen.

The cord-clamping procedure is now usually delayed for a couple of minutes, until the cord stops pulsating and becomes cool and limp. The blood in the cord is the baby's blood. By waiting until the cord stops pulsating before he cuts it, the doctor can give the baby as much as 75 cc. of blood that would otherwise have flowed onto the floor of the delivery room. The cord is not milked; the blood is allowed to flow into the baby at its own rate. Although studies even in the late 1940s showed this to be a benefit in preventing iron-deficiency in babies, some obstetricians may still clamp the cord right after delivery, unless parents object.

The baby is usually placed on the abdomen of his mother, who is usually semi-sitting. However, she may still have to ask that this be done. Her body, with a covering blanket over both mother and baby, provides adequate warmth, although delivery rooms are still usually cooled for the obstetrician's comfort. Gone is the custom of holding the baby up by the heels to "drain the mucus," thus suddenly straightening a spine that has been curved for months. This was done until recently, especially for drugged babies, to help wake them up.

The cord, no longer pulsating and warm to the touch, is clamped about two inches from the baby. Another clamp is placed about three inches away on the mother's side of the cord. The clamps look like home-permanent curlers. For a home birth, boiled white shoe strings may be used. The cut is made with scissors between the two clamps. There are no nerve fibers in the cord, and no pain is involved. The stump on the baby is sometimes trimmed to half an inch or so by the nurse. The cord could be left long. Actually, there is, in theory, no requirement that the cord be cut at all. However, the crib would be rather crowded with the baby, the non-functioning cord, and the placenta. Within a few days the cord stump blackens and falls off the baby. The later appearance of the navel has no relationship to the manner of clamping and cutting of the cord.

## APGAR SCORE

First developed by a pediatrician of the same name to assess newborn health, the score requires that the obstetrician check newborn color, respiration, muscle tone, and reflexes at one minute and five minutes after birth. It may be done perfunctorily, as the assessment is fairly subjective. Points are given on a scale of 1 to 10. "All mine are nine-ten," says an obstetrician of jocular good humor. Newer scales are being developed. Also, now parents can see for themselves their baby's color and responsiveness. They can see their baby draw the first breath.

## THE DELIVERY OF THE PLACENTA

The placenta, or afterbirth, usually arrives within minutes of the birth, as the shrinking uterus prevents it from continuing to adhere to the uterine wall. The contracting uterus pushes it out, and the womb shrinks to the size of a grapefruit.

If the woman kneels or gets up on her knees instead of lying down, the afterbirth may come out more easily. She may or may not feel the contraction. Many couples are even unaware of the exit of the placenta.

There is some question as to how long one should wait for the placenta to appear. Traditionally, obstetricians have preferred that it appear almost immediately. Perhaps there is a problem. It is conceivable that the placenta has grown into the uterine wall and will not come out and a hysterectomy will be required. Perhaps the cervix could even close before the placenta exits. If so, anesthesia would be given before manual extraction. If there has been gas, spinal, saddle block, or epidural anesthesia, the placenta may have to be removed by the obstetrician because a) the anesthesia will prevent the uterus from contracting, at least not with any efficiency, and b) the woman is lying flat on her back. In such cases, the doctor reaches in and extracts the placenta by hand. If many of his patients do have more than local anesthesia, the obstetrician may become accustomed to removing the placenta himself and sees no reason to wait. Manual removal results in extra bleeding, however, and occasionally it does not come out all in one piece.

## THE POSTPARTUM INTRAVENOUS PITOCIN

The IV Pitocin after the birth is one of the procedures hardest to refuse, and there is usually less interest in refusing it after the birth because the parents are involved with the new baby. They are no longer in a frame of mind to object to hospital practices.

The IV Pitocin can cause some pain from the contracting uterus, some immobility, and can be an annoyance. To some women, it is a reminder of the medicalized birth they don't want. It is even used in normal unanesthetized birth in situations where there are adequate attendants to be with her after birth to check that the uterus remains contracted and that there is no heavy bleeding.

Physicians feel legally liable if postpartum Pitocin is not used. However, they do concede that there were years of general anesthesia and spinals when there was not this routine procedure. It is also true that if much Pitocin has been used during labor, the drug may be less effective used postpartum than it would otherwise have been. If there are twins, the Pitocin must not be used until the second twin is out.

In some of the newer birth centers and at home births, IV Pitocin postpartum is not routine. Each situation is adjudged individually, and careful postpartum observation is the rule. Sometimes there is a gush of unexplained blood, in which case the IV offers some reassurance.

Another procedure that can be extremely painful may also be done at this time. This is the prodding and rough massage of the uterus to encourage its contraction. Fingers are dug in hard above the pubic bone, often without warning. The procedure, however, can be justified because of the importance of getting all of the placenta and all clots out to prevent later bleeding. The woman should be warned ahead of time. A firm, deep pressure need not be made as painful as it is.

The nursing baby helps the uterus to contract, because breast-feeding causes the woman's body to produce its own pitocin. Massage of the uterus and even firm pressure may also be important, but sometimes the way it is done appears unnecessarily brutal. Women may prefer to massage and hold the uterus themselves. If all of the placenta has delivered, the uterus is small and firm, and bleeding is minimal, there may be no need for this procedure, only checking during the first couple of hours and occasionally thereafter.

## INFANT WARMERS

There are several types. Infrared warmers are widely used in the delivery room. Originally this special equipment and incubators were used because of prematurity or other problems. The isolation of all newborns in a nursery crib or incubator for a twelve-hour period of "observation" is also common. In this case, newborns are put in the nursery and unable to be fed or be taken to their mothers until the babies "recover" or "stabilize." The period known as "observation" is frequently a misnomer, but the term offered reassurance for many parents. Gradually this practice is disappearing. But there are still warmers in the delivery room.

Delivery room temperatures are in the low sixties, for the comfort of physicians and because of the presence of combustible gas anesthesia. The low sixties temperature is too cold for babies, even though some people used to think that the cold helped to stimulate the breathing of drugged newborns.

The use of warmers can encourage the rapid cutting of the cord to get babies off the delivery table and to a warmer place. Thus, cold delivery rooms can encourage separation of mother and baby and immediate cord clamping. This can place problems in the way of immediate breast-feeding. It is also opposed to the newer gentle Leboyer birth method.

The decision that all babies should be artificially warmed for the first few hours used to be made because their body temperatures dropped from slightly over 99° to 97° immediately after birth. A study then showed that within the first fifteen minutes after birth the temperature of all newborns drops approximately two degrees Fahrenheit, regardless of the environmental temperature. However, the warmers stayed.

The infant warmers are criticized because they prevent both body and eye contact for the newborn. Bonding is inhibited. The heat penetrates the superficial layers of the skin. Some opinion strongly suggests a relationship between the dry heat of the infant warmers and infant dehydration and consequent jaundice, now a relatively common newborn condition requiring extra fluids. In fact, the warmers double the fluid requirements for infants.

Birth rooms are generally warmer than delivery rooms. After delivery the baby is usually placed on the mother's warm body, with mother and baby both covered by a cotton blanket.

## ROUTINE INFANT SUCTIONING

Some babies who have excess fluid in their mouths are suctioned only by a rubber bulb syringe of the type found in many homes. This syringe may be used at home births. Undrugged newborns have good gag and cough reflexes, and they may be encouraged to swallow these fluids instead of having them drawn out by applying the syringe to nostrils and throat, since throat tissues are easily damaged in that way.

In many hospitals, every baby, regardless of the situation, receives routine deep suctioning. This is done by introducing a small tube into each nostril and down into the throat. "It's precautionary. It also stimulates them to breathe," parents are told. For babies, it is not a comfortable procedure. They struggle and cry. ("If they didn't, we'd know there was something wrong.") For hospital staff, it is a reassurance that if there is a breathing problem they did all that they could to clear the airways. Unprepared parents often mistakenly see it as an indication of a problem with their baby.

However, an indication for doing this procedure would be the presence of the baby's intestinal contents (meconium) in the amniotic fluid. To prevent possible aspiration of the fluid into the baby's lungs and a resulting pneumonia, the baby should be suctioned in this case.

## SILVER NITRATE

Silver nitrate in newborn eyes has been mandated by most state health departments for two generations. Its purpose is to prevent possible blindness by gonorrhea, which could be contracted as the infant passes through a birth canal infected by the gonococcus. The difficulty of ascertaining the health status of patients up to the moment of labor has resulted in continuing this regulation. It is even required for Cesarean babies who have not passed through the birth canal, since state laws do not differentiate between abdominal and vaginal birth.

A 1 percent silver nitrate solution is used, usually dispensed in individual disposable packages. It may or may not be washed out immediately with sterile water. Some babies get more of the solution than others, depending on the way it is put into the eye or dropped onto it.

All parental objections are usually met with:

a) It's a state regulation.

b) There are problems with antibiotic ointments, too.

**c)** It's too hard to check up on individual situations regarding gonorrhea.

**d)** Why *not* do it?

The problem for babies and parents is that the procedure often produces chemically induced eye irritation. The baby does not see well or open its eyes as it would without the irritation. Babies' eyes often look pink and puffy for a couple of days, to the point where the uninitiated think that newborn eyes are just naturally puffy. In fact, with silver nitrate a genuine problem with the baby's eyes can easily be overlooked.

It is now recognized that newborns can see and hear well at birth. They focus best at a distance of about sixteen inches, the distance from the infant's to mother's face when the baby is held to the breast. Bright lights and silver nitrate can inhibit visual stimulation during the early days.

Many parents request that the drops be delayed from one to four hours until their baby has had a chance to see and they have been able to have a period of eye contact with their babies. Babies born at home seldom receive silver nitrate drops because the regulation mandates the compliance of hospitals, not parents.

The American Academy of Pediatrics and the U. S. Center for Disease Control in 1981 revised their recommendations for newborn treatment for gonorrheal infection of the eyes. The former recommendation of 1 percent silver nitrate was challenged in the courts in Wisconsin and elsewhere. California, Oregon, and New York have been the first states to change their policy, but many doctors and hospitals are unaware of this. The recommendation is that 1 percent silver nitrate be used or a single dose of 1 percent tetracycline or 0.6 percent erythromycin. No agent is to be used to flush out the medication. Newborn gonorrheal infection of the eyes is to be treated with intramuscular penicillin.

# NURSING ON THE DELIVERY TABLE OR BIRTH BED

At first the request to breast-feed on the delivery table was the only way to see the new baby for more than a minute. It was a "medical decision" regardless of the health of the newborn, and could only be done if the obstetrician gave permission. Now nursing on the delivery table is generally available. However, there may be pressure to wait a few minutes until professional procedures are completed.

The nursing has no bearing on the suturing the obstetrician may be doing. Often he cannot even see the woman and baby as he sits on his stool behind drapes in the traditional delivery room.

If the baby is put to breast, he may nurse immediately. A few minutes or longer may be required before he starts, though, especially if the birth has not been gentle and the room is noisy. The purpose of immediate nursing is the comfort and reassurance it offers both baby and parents. There is no milk at this point, perhaps only a little yellowish colostrum with its protein and antibodies, but the nursing is an indication of normal newborn response and function. It also encourages the baby to swallow any fluids or mucus in his mouth and throat. For the mother, it encourages the uterus to return to its normal size because it stimulates production of the maternal oxytoxic hormone similar to pitocin, and it encourages early coming in of the milk supply.

## LEBOYER AND BONDING

The Leboyer method described in Chapter Two as synonymous with "Gentle Birth" facilitates the bonding of parents and baby. After natural childbirth became accepted, attention came to be directed also toward more humane treatment of the newborn. The question of how to implement the new concepts arose.

"We have no warm water on the labor floor," said a supervisor of a large hospital, thereby giving the lie to the hot-water requirement for birth alluded to in song and story. Other typical nurse's comments were:

"We can't see the color of the baby if we turn off the spotlight."

"Who will do the Leboyer bath? The doctors don't want to do it."

"The baby will slide off the mother's abdomen."

"We haven't the time."

"We have to do the suctioning and tagging."

"We have nothing to say about when obstetricians clamp the cord. You tell them."

Leboyer described the typical reception of the newborn as assaultive. There may be forceps, interruption of oxygen by cord clamping, noise, bright lights, cool, dry air, hard surfaces, rough handling, unsupported limbs, and hours of isolation far from nurturing human contact.

In a gentle birth, a baby may be gently massaged on its mother's abdomen, the curve of her abdomen allowing the baby's back to remain curved instead of arched. Warm water and warm skin replace cold air and a dry, rough cloth. The so-called engrossment of parents and baby with each other can now take place. It is an awesome moment when parents and offspring first look into each other's eyes.

The father may give the bath. Or this may be replaced entirely by massage on the abdomen if the parents do not wish the protective creamy vernix on the baby's skin to be washed off. Leboyer births are generally available almost everywhere, especially upon request. However, at times there is a touch of irony. After the warm water, low lights, and massage, business may suddenly resume as usual. The baby is suctioned. He or she is tagged. The silver nitrate is put in the eyes. The baby goes in the warmer. The noise level picks up. The baby is trundled off to the nursery. For a time Leboyer births were even occasionally followed by a delivery room circumcision.

Birth evolved as a medical event to occur in hospitals under the management of surgically trained people. Principles of psychology and sociology were not considered. At best they were frills in the serious business of saving lives. Anesthetized women and babies were in no condition to bond anyway. Now, however, bonding opportunities are generally available. Bonding is not a reimbursable procedure as are drugs, IVs, and anesthesia; but due to pressure from parents and the home birth movement many hospitals provide opportunity for bonding. The idea is simply that parents and babies should be together after birth.

Bonding, imprinting, engrossment between parent and young have been amply described for many years in psychological literature. Scientist Karl Lorenz discovered that newly hatched ducklings followed the first moving object they saw as they came out of the shell, including Dr. Lorenz. If animals were separated from their young at birth for minutes, even, the delicate equilibrium was found to be so disrupted that the parent could not "claim" the young.

In hospital birth the long-held assumption was that the health of mother and baby was best served by separation immediately after birth. Both needed "rest" and "recovery," it was believed. The baby saw only the ceiling and heard sounds distorted from within the plastic box, as described by the pediatrician Robert Berg. The mother was often left alone with no one in the room for long intervals. The father's presence was intermittent and uncertain. This organization of care not only separated family members, but effectively reduced public input into maternity care services. Parents didn't know what was happening to their infants; husbands didn't know what was happening to their wives.

Kennell and Klaus wrote a book, *Maternal and Infant Bonding*, that caused many to recognize the need for bonding of mother, father, infant, and even siblings. Later family follow-up was done that showed prolonged benefits of bonding, as measured by type and amount of physical contact, time spent in communication, and eye contact between parent and child.

Kennell and Klaus also described the behavior of mother and infant after birth. Without conscious thought, the mother often aligns her face with the infant's and makes eye contact. Vocalizations between mother and baby frequently are part of the interaction. Parents' touching of the newborn also tends to follow certain patterns.

Even if the baby should need oxygen or suctioning, this bonding can still occur. Parents are usually welcome in special-care nurseries, as well as regular nurseries. Nurseries may contain chairs for parents so they can touch and hold even premature babies.

The expressiveness of the faces of mother, baby, and father after birth can be unforgettable. Those who attend a non-clinically oriented birth frequently find that details of the experience remain vivid for years.

# Chapter Six

# AFTER-DELIVERY PROCEDURES

The cord-clamping, cord-cutting, and possible transfer of the baby to a crib, warmer, or incubator can occur within seconds after birth. Routine suctioning, immediate application of silver nitrate drops to the baby's eyes, the delivery of the placenta, and the postpartum IV Pitocin can occur so quickly that they have been included in the chapter on delivery. Some of these procedures might be better delayed—or avoided entirely in many cases.

Of all the routine procedures to be avoided after delivery, there is consensus among childbirth education experts that the immediate separation of baby and parents can be most harmful. Whether or not this separation contributes to obvious postpartum depression, both baby and parents, if separated, start with an adverse circumstance to overcome. If the baby should be premature or ill, the need for parental contact may be greater, not lesser. Even Cesarean birth does not require family separation. But later efforts by parents and staff can overcome the initial handicap of loss of opportunity for bonding after birth.

Long-term effects resulting from the way birth is handled are being studied. The interest has even entered the political arena. In California the legislature has appointed a panel to hold hearings on childbirth, bonding, nutrition, and early developmental experiences in an attempt to link a later tendency toward violence to these factors. The suggestion has been made that gentle approaches to childbirth might even be a start in curbing violence in society.

In the meantime, when selecting a hospital, couples should ask questions about what happens after birth as well as before birth.

## ROOMING-IN PROGRAMS

These are arrangements allowing mothers, fathers, and babies to room together in the hospital or other birthing facility. This option may be seen as only ordinary, but its achievement involved a long struggle.

Increasingly, there is no valid reason to prohibit siblings from also rooming with the parents and baby, especially in private rooms. However, a few hospitals still adhere to the old public health regulation prohibiting any visitors under the age of fourteen.

Rooming-in is generally available to almost everyone. Sometimes, however, it starts later than is optimal, the rationale being to let the mother recover from her spinal or epidural and to allow the baby to "stabilize." Some parents bring a written statement to the hospital that at no time is the baby to be taken away without their consent, that all infant care is to be done in their presence at the bedside, or that one or both parents will accompany the infant.

Rooming-in began on a small scale in the 1950s. For many years it was considered extraordinary to want to be with one's baby immediately after the birth, and even outright dangerous. It was seen as a throwback to an earlier time when newborns were placed in bed beside the mother, and little babies' cribs remained in the parents' bedroom. Freudian theory, even, was mustered to describe as "unhealthy" mothers' unwillingness to be separated from their babies. After rooming-in was introduced at Yale in the fifties, some other hospitals began to add one or two private rooming-in rooms. Insistent couples could seek them out, but they were seldom advertised. Then there might be a forty-eight-hour waiting period after delivery for rooming-in.

Increased numbers of prepared couples having natural childbirth made the old central nurseries appear obsolete. Mothers' requests to have access to their babies was only reasonable, especially as the incidence of breast-feeding began to rise in parents of a higher socioeconomic class.

Even so, objections were raised. What would the nursery nurses do if the babies were not in the nursery? Nursery nurses were unaccustomed to going into postpartum rooms except briefly to deliver babies for brief, widely spaced feedings. Then again, women needed their sleep. Babies needed to be observed. The fathers would bring germs.

Babies who had been in their mothers' rooms for longer than the prescribed feeding times, or who had been touched by fathers were not always able to return to the nursery, although the reasoning behind this was unclear. Babies born out of hospital in cars or planes were also banished from the nursery as being "contaminated." Strangely, ill babies, babies who had been in patients' rooms, or babies born out of hospital could be found frequently in isolated laundry or utility rooms, near the nursery, but not in it. Infection had been a continued concern of hospitals to the point of closing certain nurseries or wings of hospitals. The problem was later determined to be related to crowding and the central nursery system of many nurses going from baby to baby. It was not because father and mother had held the baby, or because babies had been in rooms longer than the usual fifteen-minute feeding periods, or had been born in the car.

Having one's baby in the room with her was often a privilege of private patients only. Some babies, especially those of clinic mothers, never went to their mothers at all during the hospital stay. The purpose was to save staff time. Bottles were propped up for the baby or given by nurses in the nursery. Breast-feeding was thus effectively denied to those mothers.

"Dry-up" pills or injections of estrogenic substances to dry up milk and prevent breast discomfort are still used for women who do not nurse. A new substance to avoid possible hazards of estrogens is now beginning to be promoted. It acts by inhibiting the secretion of the female hormone prolactin. Side effects include lowered blood pressure and feelings of weakness, which hardly seem a plus with a new baby to care for, and long-term effects are not known. Prolactin circulating in the blood is believed to have a calming effect on women.

Some people still wonder whether women are too ill and tired, as a result of the rigors of birth, to be interested and able to care for their babies. Can they be trusted to observe their babies? This latter question overlooks the fact that nursery care has always consisted largely of diaper changes every four hours and distribution of babies to mothers for feeding. Nurses do not stand over babies in a constant watch, as many have fantasized. Hospital nurseries function mainly as holding areas.

The several types of rooming-in include twenty-four-hour rooming-in, except as parents wish to return the baby to the nursery. In another type, babies may be taken out of the nursery during the day, but returned at night with parents' instructions to bring the baby if he wakes and cries, or if the mother feels engorged with milk. In practice, the different types tend to merge, as parents decide when to leave off babies at the nursery and when to retrieve them. Babies may go to the nursery if there are visitors, or the baby may remain in the room, especially if the visitors are family members.

A major benefit of rooming-in is the ability to establish an effective breast-feeding relationship with the baby. The old four-hour feeding schedules have been made obsolete by research which at least is thirty-five years old. Hunger in babies is felt as pain because the stomach contracts suddenly rather than gradually as in adult hunger. Withholding night feedings does not teach babies to "sleep through." The infant's sucking encourages milk production. Even the presence of the baby, especially in the early days, stimulates the let-down of milk. With rooming-in, parents can be assured that the baby is comfortable and not crying behind glass in another room.

Rooming-in babies are usually quiet because their needs for milk and comfort are better met. Also, parents decide about visitors, and plan when and whom to invite instead of having unexpected visitors dropping by anytime during visiting hours.

## VITAMIN K

Although many parents have been unaware of it, vitamin K has been given routinely to newborns for at least a couple of generations. Parents are not often present to observe or comment about it, and they do not sign a special consent as they would for circumcision.

The purpose is to encourage blood-clotting. For a few days after birth, babies are not able to produce vitamin K in their bodies, although within a week intestinal bacteria begin to synthesize the vitamin. Therefore, if surgery such as circumcision is contemplated within the first week, then the injection of vitamin K may have its use.

Perhaps babies of malnourished women receiving inadequate protein and not eating leafy green vegetables that contain vitamin K may benefit from vitamin K, especially after a forceps delivery, which might produce cerebral bleeding. Most hospital staff are unaware of why the vitamin is being given. It might help, so why not do it?

The following objections have been raised to the routine administration of vitamin K soon after birth:

a) The injection disturbs the baby.

b) Early circumcision is not a justifiable reason. Many feel that early circumcision, too, is in opposition to the concept of gentle birth. Moreover, the injection is given to girl babies also.

c) The research is inadequate, but it appears that vitamin K, along with Pitocin, is associated with the development of newborn jaundice, which is discussed immediately below. There seems to be no real interest in researching this connection adequately.

d) The dosage is also being questioned. A nurse states, "I think small babies get jaundice more frequently than larger babies because I have to give the same dose to five-pounders as to eight-pounders."

Only parents can refuse this procedure. Nurses must follow orders. Many physicians, fearing censure or malpractice, do not feel comfortable not ordering vitamin K for all babies, or even see why there should be any objection.

## JAUNDICE AND BILILIGHTS

Increasing numbers of babies, perhaps one or two in every hospital nursery, may be observed lying naked with bandaged eyes under fluorescent lights for phototherapy.

Jaundice is an accumulation of yellow bile (bilirubin) in the blood. Bilirubin is derived from the breakdown of hemoglobin, which is present in red blood cells. The skin and eyes may appear yellowish if the bilirubin count is high.

Jaundice in the adult is caused by disease or obstruction of the bile duct. In the newborn, it is almost always caused by immaturity of the system that metabolizes hemoglobin during the first week or two of life.

Newborns have more hemoglobin than adults because during prenatal life more is needed by the infant to assure sufficient oxygen. Red blood cells have a life-span of about 120 days in an adult, 70 days in the newborn. The breakdown products at the end of this life-span are metabolized and excreted. Intestinal bacteria, which appear after the baby begins to eat, as well as liver enzymes aid in metabolizing these substances.

Some bilirubin is bound to protein molecules called albumin, and some is unbound. The unbound can cause problems because it diffuses into tissues and is toxic. Most present tests do not discriminate between the two types.

Both prevention and treatment of newborn jaundice involves frequent feedings and providing light on the baby's skin. Rarely, transfusion is required. The light used may be daylight through a glass window or it may be brief exposures even to direct sunlight. Artificial light from the blue part of the spectrum is also used.

As with other childbirth procedures, there are connections among after-delivery procedures. One intervention, whether necessary or routine, may require another procedure. For example, factors other than wrapping babies and feeding them on schedule may affect the incidence of newborn jaundice.

The use of diuretics during pregnancy can also increase the risk of newborn jaundice. Diuretics during pregnancy may be given for fluid retention without recognition that there is a normal increase in blood supply and tissue fluids at that time. These babies may be more vulnerable to jaundice. Babies who are placed in the warmer after birth may lose body fluids from the infrared radiant dry heat, as mentioned in Chapter Five. Both dehydration from the radiant warmers in the delivery room and inadequate number of feedings because of "feeding schedules" contributes to the problem, as mentioned above.

Many childbirth professionals and parents feel that vitamin K almost certainly has an association with jaundice and would like to see this researched instead of being accepted without question as a ritual of birth. The use of Pitocin during birth is also associated with the development of jaundice, but the reasons are not clear.

A high bilirubin count may be unavoidable. The total serum bilirubin is measured in milligrams per hundred milliliters. The average is 6 for full-term babies, and premature babies' levels peak at 10–12. The information frequently given to these parents is, "If the count gets to 20, there could be brain damage."

The need to obtain frequent blood samples from babies' heels to monitor the bilirubin count virtually assures that babies will get regular, perhaps daily, heel sticks. These heel sticks are painful. Babies may be separated from their mothers and even removed from the breast if the count gets too high. The mother may not be able to leave the hospital with the baby until the count goes down. Separation from parents at this important time can interfere with parent-baby attachment and cause parental anxiety. If bililights are needed, parents need to be prepared ahead of time for the sight of seeing their three-day-old infant under bililights, apparently ill when they thought they had a healthy baby. The baby, with bandaged eyes to prevent eye damage from the lights, also loses the visual stimulation especially important during the early days. To avoid this, parents should spend as much time as possible with the baby, giving verbal and touch stimulation. The lights can be brought into the parent's room.

The exposure of newborns to blue-tinted lights to hasten bilirubin destruction has been described as risky because this phototherapy may transform bilirubin into other toxic substances. Blood exchange, a technique where the infant's blood is replaced with transfused blood, is inherently dangerous, although life-saving in certain instances of blood incompatibility. One percent of the infant's blood supply may be required for diagnosis by the heel sticks, and furthermore, the test is subject to error. A new machine, however, has been developed that requires less blood and gives results in ten to fifteen minutes.

Also, not all bilirubin is harmful; only the free bilirubin unattached to albumin is dangerous, as free bilirubin could reach the infant's brain and disrupt the delicate connections still forming among nerve cells. The new machine will determine the amount of unbound bilirubin, more important than the total count now obtained.

The fear of being unable to refuse hospital procedures surrounding the bilirubin count, combined with diagnostic uncertainties, has led some parents to comment, "After you have your baby, it's better to leave immediately or within a few hours before the count goes up. Pick up your baby and get the hell out of there." If parents do leave soon after birth, as many do, the baby can be brought to the pediatrician's office for the test. If the count is high, the baby can be nursed frequently and the infant's skin exposed to daylight through glass. This may be adequate light exposure.

The factors previously mentioned—vitamin K, Pitocin, lack of light on the skin, infrequent feedings—affect the bilirubin count. Other factors are prematurity (which decreases the level of albumin protein available for binding and hampers the body's ability to process and excrete bilirubin) and a difference in blood type between the mother and baby (which may, rarely, require transfusion). Certain drugs used during pregnancy such as injected Valium, Aspirin, hydrocortisone, and thiazide diuretics may also be factors in newborn jaundice, also sulfa drugs and erythromycin.

At the same time, there is inadequate study of both the effects of prolonged maternal fasting during labor and the relationship of vitamin K and Pitocin to the development of jaundice, as well as the effects of the continuous dry heat of infant warmers. Some nurseries may have no windows. The fluorescent lights used to break down the excess bilirubin may also cause destruction of essential vitamins such as riboflavin. For this reason, some physicians suggest that babies under the lights be given vitamin supplements.

The jaundice just described is called physiologic jaundice. Rarely (in one of two hundred infants), breast milk may be a cause. In these cases, there appears to be a substance in breast milk that inhibits liver enzyme activity. Frequently, the physiologic jaundice is confused with breast-milk jaundice, and the baby is removed from the breast. When this happens, the count does indeed go down from its peak at three to four days, but in most cases it would go down anyway.

In breast-milk jaundice the rise in bilirubin occurs, not during the first few days, but during the second week, when the baby is at home. The level may reach 20 in the third week of life with no apparent danger, unlike the situation with the unbound bilirubin of physiologic jaundice. The baby is lively and has good appetite. If the bilirubin does continue to rise, the baby may have to be fed a formula for a day or two while the mother pumps or hand expresses her milk to maintain the supply, but does not give it to the baby. Women in this situation should talk with childbirth educators or La Leche League leaders for advice in pumping and expressing.

It is difficult or impossible for many women to pump milk soon after the birth, but at least the breast receives some stimulation in this way, to help maintain the milk supply. The mother should remember that except for these rare cases, her milk is not harmful to her baby and she may continue to breast feed.

However, because breast-milk jaundice is so rare there are almost no testing facilities. To be on the safe side, according to their view, unfortunately many physicians automatically assume that all newborn jaundice is breast-milk jaundice and suggest that all babies with a high bilirubin count be removed from the breast temporarily. Not everyone agrees with this recommendation.

Discontinuing breast-feeding does not help physiologic jaundice, but, as said previously, misinformation results in many babies being removed unnecessarily from the breast. Some are removed permanently, as discouragement, fear, and the difficulty of pumping milk in the early days take their toll. Breast infections may occur if nursing is stopped and the breasts are not emptied.

## SUGAR WATER

Some hospitals strongly encourage the use of sugar water, or plain water in some facilities when parents object to sugar water, at every feeding. The purpose is to increase the amount of water in the babies' system, but this practice also acts to delay the coming in of an ample milk supply because the baby sucks less often and less strongly. Also, the bottle requires a different kind of sucking, which can confuse the baby. If given the opportunity, babies may nurse eight to ten or more times a day on the second or third day when the milk is in. Uninformed people may think that the baby is eating "too often" and is therefore "not getting enough." As a result, babies may be shortchanged on sucking opportunities or given formula.

Babies are born with a desire to suck even if the milk is not in. The frequent opportunity to suck is a factor in bringing in an early milk supply, even as soon as the second day. If the baby is placed in the mother's bed after birth, as is possible in some hospitals, the baby may nurse almost constantly at times. If the baby is at least in the same room, this may also be possible. Babies of well-nourished women are born well hydrated and do not need to eat anything before the milk comes in. In the days before prepared childbirth and breast-feeding most hospitals did not offer formula to the drugged babies for the first day anyway, and the babies were often limited to two feedings the second day. After that, they got only five feedings a day and none during the night because mothers were tired and babies, it was thought, should "learn to sleep through the night." Fortunately, those days are over.

Bottles of sugar water may be offered to every baby in many hospitals to combat the possibility of jaundice or even to raise the baby's blood sugar level, which may have dropped as a result of prolonged maternal fasting during labor, regardless of the fact that this also delays the coming in of the milk and acts to reduce the mother's milk supply. Sometimes babies are given sugar water in the nursery, or even pacifiers, and parents are not informed.

## THE BREAST AND BREAST-FEEDING

### *The Breast*

The milk is formed, not near the surface of the breast, but near the chest wall. In the breast, the alveoli, or small spaces looking like bunches of grapes, are lined with milk-secreting cells. Sixteen or twenty ducts carry the milk down to small sinuses, or spaces,

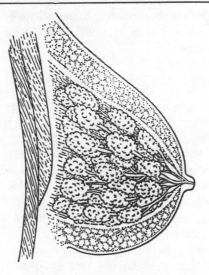

*The Breast, showing the alveoli*

behind the nipple. Milk is constantly being formed. The breast does not "fill" every three to four hours, as some have believed.

The let-down reflex acts to constrict the alveoli and send the milk down the ducts, resulting in a tingling sensation for the lactating woman. The let-down reflex is initiated most likely by stimulation of nerve endings in the nipple. The neuro-hormonal impulse stimulates the pituitary gland to produce oxytocin. The oxytocin constricts the alveoli of the breast to squeeze milk down the ducts. Sucking, or even the mother simply seeing a hungry baby, may initiate the reflex, as may the sound of a crying baby even in another room. Orgasm may also set it in motion.

The more frequently the reflex is activated, the greater the supply of milk. The supply is increased by ample fluid and nutrient intake, and by confidence as opposed to fear.

Breast-feeding does not result in an altered contour of the breasts or sagging breasts. Breast size may increase temporarily, however, and support is recommended.

The amount of milk is not related to the size of the breast nor the age of the mother. The size of the breast is determined by fatty tissue, not by milk-producing tissue. Virtually all women can nurse. Twins can be totally breast-fed if the couple has information and encouragement.

## *Breast-feeding*

Breast-feeding is a process, not a procedure. Information is needed by both parents immediately at birth, and before.

Breast-feeding has become more the norm than the exception, beginning in 1970, when prepared childbirth became accepted at an ever-increasing rate, as more couples learned about it and demanded it, and as couples became comfortable with birth and didn't want to miss out on this experience as had so many of their parents. Breast-feeding was taught in childbirth classes and the national organization for breast-feeding, La Leche League, became ever more active. Nursing almost automatically followed natural childbirth as the baby was born and handed to the mother who put her child to breast right on the delivery table.

During the mid-sixties, Eva Salber, M.D., a Harvard School of Public Health epidemiologist, had found that breast-feeding prevalence was greatest among higher socioeconomic and educated couples, but, as with prepared childbirth, other groups began to breast feed. In 1970 only 5.5 percent of U.S. mothers were still breast-feeding after six months, but by 1979, 28 percent were still breast-feeding after that time, which is the time of the most rapid infant growth and highest nutritional needs. Currently, many women nurse for a year or two, even though the toddler nurses less often and, of course, eats other food.

The American Academy of Pediatrics has found a lower incidence of infant illness, lessened risk of allergy, and many other benefits for breast-fed babies, and has strongly endorsed breast-feeding. The result has been fewer comments, even in formula advertising, that formula is "as good as mother's milk." There are also fewer questions from friends and relatives such as, "When are you going to give him *real* food?"

During the past few years infant formula companies have been expanding their markets into the third-world countries. When infant formula is provided in a clinical setting during the early days of life, women's milk dries up and they become dependent on formula. Because it's expensive, they water it down at times to make it last. Lack of refrigeration facilities also threatens infant health when bottle feeding is introduced.

For the mother, breast-feeding encourages rapid recovery from childbirth and lessened bleeding because of its effect of contracting the uterus. The post-birth "period," called the lochia, lasting two to three weeks as the discharge turns from red to brown and then to a yellowish discharge, is shortened by breast-feeding. Studies have shown a more rapid return to sexual interests among breast-feeding mothers, although the reasons are not entirely clear.

Breast-feeding also tends to inhibit ovulation, especially if no formula or solids are offered, although this is not considered a reliable form of contraception. The diaphragm is frequently the contraception method of choice for breast-feeding women, since birth-control pills inhibit milk production besides having uncertain effects on the baby. "I breast fed my male child fourteen months while on oral contraceptives. He got female hormones. No one told me," one woman says.

Breast-feeding women have a lower incidence of fibrocystic disease and probably of breast cancer also, though most studies are not designed to demonstrate this since the definition of a "breast-feeding mother" varies from one who breast feeds for one week to years.

Toddlers may be offered "comfort nursing" a time or two each day. Some women do "tandem nursing" breast-feeding two children of different ages, although both children may not be on the breast at the same time.

Weaning is gradual, depending on mother, the child, and circumstances. Sudden weaning is hard on the child and uncomfortable, or even painful, for the woman whose breasts may become full and hard when the child does not nurse.

An approving or disapproving husband has a profound effect on breast-feeding. Does he see her achievement as worthwhile? Will he work with her to overcome difficulties? The self-esteem of both parents can be raised as they watch their child grow on the milk she produces.

HOW TO BREAST FEED

The baby, to have access to the milk, must be put all the way on the breast, including the area surrounding the nipple, known as the areola. The baby's jaws come together on the milk-containing sinuses behind the nipple. A tentative approach is more likely to produce sore breasts as the baby frantically chews on the nipple. However, the baby's face must not be pressed into the breast so that the nose is blocked and the baby must struggle away from the breast to get air. When removing the baby from the breast, using a finger to depress the breast helps to break the suction. Pulling the baby off is hard both on the infant and the nipples.

Both breasts are used each time the baby is fed. Sometimes "three-sided" nursing is helpful. The first breast is used for several minutes, then the second breast, then back to the first one. This can give extra breast stimulation for nursing and a small amount of additional milk.

The question has always been, Who is responsible for breast-feeding? The obstetrician is responsible for the breast and its diseases. The pediatrician is responsible for advice on infant feeding. Nurses also exert strong influence over hospital patients by their attitudes and the information they give. Childbirth educators and the La Leche League have been largely responsible for educating hospital personnel and parents. Many questions arise after the return home, therefore the need for community resource information. Some informed nurses have encouraged parents to call the hospital if there are later problems. Childbirth educators and La Leche League leaders usually offer the most accurate and comprehensive information. Breast-feeding, like childbirth, is a skill to be learned.

The La Leche League was organized in 1957 by parents in response to the realization that accurate information on breast-feeding was not readily available. As in other childbirth organizations, parent and medical leadership have combined. The organization headquarters provides research information and support for local La Leche chapters nationwide. A four-session series of meetings is offered before the birth, and trained counselors work with parents and hospitals without charge on a twenty-four-hour telephone basis. Women may attend meetings and afterward to talk with other breast-feeding women. The contribution La Leche makes to parenting and breast-feeding is great. When parents move to a new area of the country, they frequently contact La Leche to become acquainted with other parents and available local childbirth facilities.

Comments of friends or relatives may be helpful, but they may also be demoralizing. "No one in our family has ever been able to nurse," "Are you sure he's gaining weight?" "Are you still nursing him?" "She would sleep better if you would feed her." Fathers of babies may be jealous of the close relationship of mother and child and consequently feel left out. If the husband acknowledges and communicates this feeling, however, it often tends to subside, and he can support his wife against ill-informed friends and relatives and protect against intrusions. Sometimes a "good" baby is erroneously defined as one who sleeps a lot and eats regularly and infrequently.

## OVERCOMING HURDLES TO BREAST-FEEDING

Most problems occur during the first two weeks, especially the first week.

An episiotomy can be a hurdle to breast-feeding because it is difficult to get into a comfortable position. The pain from a sore bottom as a result of an episiotomy is not conducive to easy milk let-down. Ice on the incision or a warm sitz bath can offer relief.

There may also be pain from the uterus as it contracts during nursing. Knowing the cause of the pain can help. The shrinking of the uterus after birth is necessary. It is a positive sign. "After pains" are common after a second or third baby even when the woman is not breast-feeding. The discomfort is often more prolonged after a second or subsequent baby, perhaps because the uterus contracts less efficiently. No one knows for sure. A hot-water bottle may feel good. Lying prone on a small pillow or hot-water bottle may help, and it aids the uterus in returning to its normal size, but this position cannot be used during nursing. Many women prefer to lie on their side to breast feed or to sit tipped slightly backward with their knees bent and resting on pillows. The baby may rest on a pillow on the mother's lap to bring the baby high enough to nurse.

*Engorgement* of the breasts can be very painful, another part of after-birth pain. In all fantasies of the possible pain associated with childbirth, few women are prepared for the experience of pain after the delivery, and few know how to minimize it. Those who nurse infrequently or not at all during the first day or so "because there is no milk" seem more likely to have this problem. Those who try to "get the baby on a schedule" seem also more likely to get engorged to the point of pain. If the breast becomes hard with the nipple pulled flat, the baby cannot latch onto the breast.

The problem is partly hormonal rather than an excess of milk. However, the milk may be started manually by massaging the breast on all quadrants from armpit to nipple before the baby is put on the breast. A warm shower may be helpful in getting the milk started and in softening the breast. Engorgement typically lasts only a few days or less as the milk comes in. Some women never get engorged. "My baby nursed at intervals all night just before the milk came in," one mother says. "She seemed to know it was almost there as though she could smell or taste it. When it gushed in she got the most contented look on her face. She really worked to get it in on that second day."

*Sore nipples* are another possibility, occurring as do other types of pain only in the early days after birth. Here are some suggestions for minimizing nipple pain, even if it cannot be avoided altogether for most women. Nurse early and frequently, but not for long at first. Get the baby all the way on the breast, not just on the nipple. Air-dry the nipples after nursing. Use no soap (the milk is sterile as it comes out) or drying lotions or disinfectants. Supportive bras, but not tight bras which constrict the breast, are best. Plastic bra liners should never be used, since they cause nipple pain and even infections. Leaking, which occurs mostly in the early days and weeks after birth, can be controlled by an old cotton handkerchief placed in the bra over the nipple. Hair dryers, sun, exposure to the warmth of a light bulb have been used to dry the nipples after feeding to prevent irritation and pain. Lanolin or vitamin E oil may be put on the nipple to prevent possible cracking and need not be washed off before the next feeding. By exposing the nipples to air and sun, and washing them with a rough washcloth during pregnancy, the mother may toughen them to prevent real soreness when the baby starts feeding.

*Flat nipples,* sometimes called "inverted" nipples, may be drawn out by the baby, or they may be drawn out manually before the birth. The use of Woolwich nipple shields, small inexpensive cups that use suction to draw the nipples out, are available from the hospital or La Leche League, and are used by many women in the first days of breast-feeding.

*Clogged ducts* are evident by a "lump" in the breast. The breast may be massaged to help correct the problem. The baby may continue to nurse. Tight clothing and infrequent nursing may be a cause.

*Breast infections* may occur early or later and are treated by rest, fluids, and maybe ampicillin from the physician. Symptoms are a warm, sore spot on the breast, perhaps a rise in body temperature. The baby must continue to nurse during the breast infection to keep the milk flowing. If soreness, nipple cracking, or an infection makes nursing on that side difficult, the milk may be hand expressed, pumped with a suction pump, or started manually before the baby is put on the breast. Infections may be prevented by keeping the hands very clean, eating well, resting, and getting plenty of fluids.

During colds and other illnesses, women can continue to nurse. The baby is not at increased risk of infection, since the mother's antibodies come through the milk. In fact, it has been well-documented that breast-fed babies have fewer and less-severe colds and infections than those on formula.

### MILK SUPPLY

When the leaking of the early days and weeks lessens, it does not mean that the milk supply is diminishing. Many parents can hardly believe the milk supply is adequate. But even twins can be nursed. However, the milk looks thin and bluish, and parents have no way to measure the amount taken. No wonder they may accept a non-nutritive fluid such as sugar water if they don't realize that it delays and inhibits milk production.

It is true that there are fewer air bubbles with a breast-fed baby than a bottle-fed baby, because the baby tends to swallow less air. Any regurgitated milk does not have as sour a smell as formula. Also, the stools of breast-fed babies do not have the unpleasant odor of those of formula-fed babies until solid foods are introduced, usually at five to six months.

Colic is infrequent in breast-fed babies because the milk curd is smaller than that of cow's milk. Colic may be due to immature digestive organs, and tends to disappear at three months of age. A calm atmosphere, feedings as frequent as the baby wishes, gentle burping, and laying the baby in varied positions, sometimes with the abdomen against a warm hot-water bottle, can help.

Weighing the baby before and after feeding is usually unwise. The information has little value even if the scales are very accurate. If the baby urinates between weighings, the reading is thrown off. More important, the milk supply varies during the day. It is less under stress, including the stress of having the measure taken by a watchful nurse, a time when it may be hard to let down milk. A contented, growing baby with a daily supply of wet diapers is the best measure of successful breast-feeding.

The mother's milk supply depends on the demand. The frequency of feeding is more important than the length, though after the soreness has passed the feedings can be more leisurely. The baby has a growth spurt at approximately six weeks and again at three months. At these times, it may be necessary temporarily to increase the number of feedings by several a day for a few days until the supply builds up to meet the new demand.

The supply builds up gradually over the early weeks. Working women can then pump milk, freeze it, and store it for baby-sitters and fathers to give by bottle. Different babies accept it from a bottle with great variability. The sucking action is different on a bottle. On the breast, rather than sucking, the baby extends the lower jaw and tongue and then brings the jaws together against the sinuses behind the nipple.

The breast-feeding woman needs an extra quart of nutritive fluids such as milk or juices and an extra meal each day, because the baby takes calories from her in the milk. Nursing, in fact, tends to encourage the return to her pre-pregnant weight without any real conscious effort if the mother avoids junk foods. A marginal weight gain during pregnancy and a limiting of food intake afterward can diminish the milk supply.

The breast-feeding woman as well as the pregnant woman needs protein, eggs, milk products, salads, several vegetables and fruits each day, and whole grain products such as wheatgerm, corn meal, and oatmeal. She should avoid excessive fats (which may inhibit the milk supply) sugar, salt, and excessive caffeine (which may make her baby restless and wakeful). Cigarette smoking is harmful to the baby before and during breast-feeding.

Breast-feeding, when desired, is easily accomplished on trains, planes, and at dinner parties or work. A two-piece outfit that can be raised from the waist is best. As the upper part is raised, the baby's body covers the bare midriff. Scarves can be draped loosely over the shoulder. Soft carriers worn on the body can be used, with the baby nursed in the carrier.

## HINDRANCES TO BREAST-FEEDING

a) Solid foods, even in small amounts, introduced in the early weeks and months inhibit sucking on the breast and therefore reduce the milk supply.

b) Growth charts, which were devised for infants on formulas and canned baby foods, give unrealistic expectations.

c) Nipple shields which cover the nipple to prevent soreness do not allow the milk to come through as well. The breast receives inadequate stimulation. Also, the baby can get accustomed to the shield and refuse to nurse without it. Woolwich shields are helpful, but their purpose is to draw out flat or inverted nipples, and they are not used during actual nursing.

d) Sugar water or plain water offered as part of the feeding plan can also inhibit nursing. The sucking on a bottle requires a different motion than that required to get milk from the breast, and sucking on the bottle can inhibit the frequent, strong sucking needed for weight gain and milk supply.

e) Insistence on limiting feedings to the 3–4 hour intervals of outmoded "schedules." This is a sure way to reduce the milk supply. Infrequent feedings mean the baby gets less to eat; the weight gain is therefore less; the breasts get inadequate stimulation to produce milk. Also, there is the erroneous assumption that the milk supply is constant throughout the twenty-four hours. In addition, the baby often cries between feedings, and when the scheduled time to feed arrives the baby may be too tired to nurse adequately. A crying baby untended makes the parents tense and fatigued, and this is no help to milk let-down.

f) Supplementary bottles. A self-fulfilling prophesy results because bottles are a way of weaning a baby from the breast, not of building up breast milk.

g) A discouraging spiel, from anyone, like the following: "You need your rest. The baby needs more fluids. Get her used to the bottle while young. Use the shield to protect your nipples. Don't nurse too often, you'll get sore. The bilirubin count is going up, we may have to take her off the breast. Let's weigh her before and after nursing. Don't get your hopes up too high, lots of women can't nurse without supplements."

h) Maternal medications which may reach the baby through the milk, such as pain medications after a Cesarean. Sometimes short-acting medication is taken immediately after a feeding to minimize infant exposure. Parents may get information on this subject from La Leche. Sometimes they may decide that pain medication can be dispensed with. Penicillin, though, is usually not a contraindication to nursing.

The benefits of breast-feeding become evident within two to three weeks. Putting the baby to breast becomes almost an automatic response to a baby in distress. It's easy. It's cheap. Nothing else is needed. There are fewer digestive problems. The baby is never allergic to mother's milk. Occasionally the baby may be sensitive to something the mother eats. Very rarely, as stated elsewhere, a case occurs of breast-milk jaundice. The baby can be fed anywhere, anyplace, and can be comforted this way for much of the first year and longer. The baby can be fed in bed without you getting up for bottles. It's comforting and relaxing for the mother as well. The baby may even "comfort nurse" on the father, sucking on his chest or shoulder, as some parents have reported.

# CIRCUMCISION

Many informed couples now question this procedure, which has become almost routine in this country, so routine that parents have actually thought this surgery is required by state law as is the silver nitrate solution for babies' eyes. A consent form is given to the mother for signature prior to this operation. In most cases it is hardly informed consent because she does not know the facts about the surgery nor why it is done. Clearly, she is expected to sign, and she usually does. The consent form becomes an inadvertent solicitation, according to some.

The surgery is done by the obstetrician, not the pediatrician. If it were to be delayed, instead of being done during the hospital stay, the pediatrician would do it.

Circumcision is virtually the only operation performed without the use of anesthesia. The two reasons given are, first, that drugs and anesthesia are harmful to newborns. (Seldom does the explanation recognize that drugs and anesthesia cross the placenta and have been given freely during labor) and secondly, that newborns "do not feel pain" or will not remember it. Anyone who is acquainted with newborns can hardly believe that they do not feel pain exquisitely. Observers of babies whose foreskin is being cut off can hardly doubt the pain and fear.

"Circ rooms" are seldom shown to prospective parents touring the hospital. They seldom have access to more than a comment or two on the subject of circumcision: "We had it done, I don't know why. We'd said no to so many things, the IV, the monitoring equipment, the episiotomy."

There are strong social pressures on physicians and families for circumcision. Yet in 1975 the American Academy of Pediatrics made a strong statement as a result of work done by its ad hoc task force on this topic: "There are no valid medical indications for circumcision in the newborn period." The American College of Obstetrics and Gynecology does not support circumcision either, but obstetricians continue to do it.

The rate of circumcision in the fifties and sixties was reported as 90–98 percent, with fewer circumcisions done in the southern part of the country. By 1980 the rate was reported as 75 percent.

Dr. James Hutchinson of the Royal College of Surgeons in England is described as the instigator of non-ritual circumcision as a preventative of masturbation. He proposed in 1891 that "if public opinion permitted their adoption—measures more radical than circumcision would be a true kindness." The Puritan heritage in America supported this "treatment." Until 1936 circumcision was a recommended "treatment" for masturbation, associated at the time with insanity, in Holt's *Diseases of Infancy and Childhood*. Until 1977 clitoridectomy for the female was covered by Blue Cross.

Before 1900 few non-Jewish children were circumcised, and at that time mild anesthesia was used. As birth moved to the hospital, however, these ways were seen as old-fashioned. Birth at home was uncivilized, breast-feeding was old-fashioned, and the foreskin was something to be gotten rid of.

The justification for circumcision developed after, not before, the operation was widely practiced. The rationale for doing it has been disproved. Circumcision has no connection with the incidence of cancer of the penis or the cervix. That assumption was made because of the low incidence of these cancers in the Jewish population. However, it was later ascertained that this is rather because of the greater stability of family relationships and less promiscuity by this part of the population. These cancers are associated with early and frequent sexual activity with multiple partners and perhaps lack of general hygiene, not with the presence of foreskin.

A reason given for circumcision soon after birth is non-retractable foreskin. However, the fact is that newborn foreskin is not retractable and should not be retracted. If an uninformed pediatrician does this, the baby will experience severe pain. Scar tissue may form causing later problems, including need for circumcision.

The surgery is not entirely without risk. Medical literature includes a long list of potential problems, although they are uncommon.

Sometimes circumcision is also thought to improve personal hygiene, implying that males cannot be taught cleanliness. Is the need for cleaning our ears a reason to lop off the outer ear?

Many parents permit the surgery because they wish their sons to look like their peers. Others feel that they will wait and let the child make the decision. If he later decides for circumcision, anesthesia can be given.

The circumcision procedure is generally as follows, although there can be variations. In a special room for this purpose, the baby is laid on his back on a molded plastic tray. His wrists are fastened down, with his arms straight and partly out to the side. His legs are drawn apart, straightened and fastened down at the ankles, a very unbabylike position on a hard surface. The crying is ignored as an expected part of the procedure. A drape is placed over the baby, leaving only the penis and the face exposed. A snip is made in the foreskin, which almost covers the head of the penis. An instrument is then inserted and moved around the head of the penis to free the foreskin. Next, a small metal bell is placed over the head of the penis, and the obstetrician pulls the stretchy, pink foreskin up around the outside of the bell. A clamp, looking like a small vise is attached. The foreskin, now between the bell and the clamp, is trimmed off with a knife like so much excess dough around the edge of a pie plate.

Gauze is placed over the penis, and the baby is then diapered and returned to the nursery at the nurse's convenience. Healing requires a few days, during which the baby should not be placed on his stomach. Urination, very frequent in the newborn, reactivates the pain and crying.

Mothers and fathers seldom know when the circumcision is done, as it is performed whenever it is convenient for the obstetrician, who wants to get it done before mother and baby leave the hospital. Therefore, babies may not be brought to their parents for comforting afterward.

Many feel that circumcision is needlessly barbaric. It could be done later, when medication could be used and the blood would clot better. One of the parents could hold the child during the procedure. He could be nursed immediately afterward. The ideas that it must be done early at any cost "because it will hurt more later" and, "the obstetrician is in the hospital so it's convenient now" should be reexamined. Both parents need to discuss their feelings and desires before birth, as after birth there is often pressure to make an immediate decision.

## LEAVING THE HOSPITAL

There is wide choice in most cases as to how long mother and baby remain in the hospital. A few stay an hour or two; others stay twelve hours; most stay three to six days. A Cesarean requires a stay of six to seven days. Parents have a say in this decision, although the obstetrician is the one who arranges for the discharge. The woman can sign herself out without permission, and probably her baby, too, unless there is jaundice or other problems, in which case the hospital can even announce plans for a court order, as has happened in at least a few instances. Many hospitals ask that a pediatrician check the baby before he or she is taken home.

Some parents are anxious to leave the hospital as soon as possible. They find the noise, lack of rest, other people's visitors, and need to conform to the routines of others to be sources of stress. They see institutional food with its white bread, its lack of fresh vegetables, and its canned fruit in sugar sauce lacking in nutrition and palatability. Breast-feeding, too, may not be encouraged by hospital routines.

Other new parents find security in the hospital. They feel that others know better than they about new babies. Women may be unsure of the help and support from their spouses at home and fear loneliness and depression. They are uncertain of grandparent relationships. Therefore, they may wish to take advantage of the hospital services as long as possible.

Decisions on when to come home depend on various factors. Obviously, the mother cannot come home right after a spinal or epidural, or if she is having more than normal bleeding or clots. If she has a catheter as a result of the spinal or epidural, or if she has soreness as a result of stitches, she may prefer to remain a hospital patient instead of taking advantage of an early discharge plan, which some hospitals now have. If the baby was premature, or severely jaundiced, or has respiratory problems, she may decide to stay in the hospital with the baby. It is hard to go home without the baby even with generous hospital visiting privileges.

If she goes home right after birth, here are some guidelines:

a) Care of episiotomy stitches. This may be limited to pouring a pitcher of water over the perineum after going to the bathroom. The stitches are usually the kind that become absorbed. If they are the kind that need to be removed, the doctor takes them out within three to four days.

b) Care of the cord stump. The stump dries and turns black, falling off after a few days. Not much needs to be done, except to avoid getting urine on it which will cause irritation. Moisture may promote infection. A bare midriff prevents the diaper from covering the cord stump.

c) Baby baths. The baby does not need to be bathed every day except for the diaper area. Babies do not ordinarily enjoy baths during the early weeks, until they gain some control over their bodies. Then one of the parents may find it easier and more enjoyable to get into the tub with the baby. Every other day with a little mild soap is adequate. Talcum powder need not be used. If shaken on, it can get into the baby's lungs. Cornstarch is a better substitute. Babies get fewer rashes with cotton clothing than with synthetics.

d) Baby's stools. These will be greenish-black and tarry at first. It is nothing to worry about. They then become more yellowish and often watery.

e) Baby care. This involves mostly feeding, holding, and comforting during the early weeks. Babies need lots of body contact. If they are in a crib, their position needs to be changed every so often because they cannot turn. It has been known for thirty years that young babies cannot be "spoiled."

f) Temperature. Newborns like a temperature of slightly over 70° F. They can easily be overdressed, however, because of plastic pants, overly snug outfits, and plastic-lined baby equipment. If their fingers and toes feel cool to the touch, they may need more warmth. If the skin feels moist and overly warm to the touch, they are too warm. For the first few days the baby's head may be covered, with blanket or cap, because much heat is lost from the head. Babies may not like bonnets with ribbons around their necks.

g) Stimulation. Babies need adequate, but not excessive stimulation from the environment. They need people, objects, and colors, but also rest and quiet.

h) Solid food. Food other than breast milk is not introduced until five to six months, as recommended by the American Academy of Pediatrics. Before that it is not only not necessary, but is not really digested. Parents may then buy baby-food grinders, to make their own baby food, instead of using the canned variety. The home-made food will be fresher, better quality, and cheaper. Ripe bananas mashed with a fork and mixed with breast milk are often used. Health-food stores often have excellent infant cereals.

i) Rest. Mother and father need rest. The woman, even though feeling fine, will spend a good part of the early days at home relaxing in bed and sleeping, maybe eating in bed and nursing in bed, because of night feedings. Baby care is mostly feeding, not work in the usual sense. Because the baby is totally dependent on the parents at first, although gradually less so, this new experience of having someone need them so totally can seem overwhelming.

j) The high-quality diet of pregnancy should be maintained for breast-feeding and recovery from childbirth. Easy-to-prepare foods should be easily available such as precooked meats, hard-boiled eggs, cheeses, fruits, raw vegetables, and milk.

k) Good posture, walking, and the exercises done prenatally, especially the pelvic rock and the Kegel exercise, help in regaining muscle tone.

Communication between the new mother and father helps to allay the possible loneliness of both parents. Her fears that he will lose interest in her or the baby, or leave all baby care to her, can be discussed. His fears that he will lose his wife's interest as she curls up on the sofa with the breast-feeding baby can be aired, too. Most couples find that sharing child-care responsibilities is best for both partners. That way, neither misses out on the experience of parenting. Neither is overburdened. Neither gets relegated to a secondary role. The couple's relationship can be stronger as a result.

The new parents should also talk about relationships with their parents. When and for how long should helping grandparents visit? Should they come at all? Should they come after the couple has lived with the new baby for a few days to establish their own parenting roles and become acquainted with the new offspring? One couple says, "We made a list of ground rules for the grandparents before they came. We recognized their need to be involved. They had missed the birth of their own children and never got to breast feed. They had been discouraged from even holding their own babies. We made sure the grandparents were included, but limited their advice and suggestions to once a day. They could give as many criticisms as they wanted during that time. We made it clear that we were the parents now, not the children. We were glad to learn from them when it did not conflict with our values. At first they could hardly take us seriously, but we persisted, and it worked beautifully. We saw a whole different dimension of them as they cooked, shopped, cleaned, and did the laundry. They respected our way of parenting. They wished they could have had some of what we had when they were parents."

# Chapter Seven

# THE CESAREAN SECTION

The rising rate of Cesarean sections is the most controversial of all practices associated with childbirth. The media have publicized this phenomenon. The federal government has become involved by the formation of a task force to explore the factors involved in the dramatic increase of Cesareans performed. Many professionals associated with childbirth feel that the number of Cesareans done is excessive. But opinions on how excessive, and for what reasons, vary. It is clear that routine obstetrical interventions play a part, and these are affected indirectly by political and economic forces.

Some obstetricians see the increase in Cesareans as progress. At least they feel a percentage of the rise may represent progress. "We are getting better babies," they say. "We're more sure of the outcome with a Cesarean. We're saving babies and preventing brain damage. Sure, the mother is uncomfortable for a while, but our interest is in getting better babies. Women are having babies later and are at greater risk, so there are more Cesareans. These are premium babies because there are fewer childbearing years left to the couple." An obstetrician teaching in a medical school asserts that in twenty years most women will deliver babies by surgery. He is one of the obstetricians who claims in print that normal birth is a dangerous process for babies. "There's a lot of force there. Babies can be battered by labor. Sometimes you get a 'toothpaste baby' squeezed out of shape. That's not good for babies. We're trying to avoid brain damage."

It is ironic that the incidence of Cesareans is rising at a time when the trend is also toward natural childbirth, patient rights, alternative birth, and midwives. Cesarean birth, the ultimate obstetrical intervention, is major abdominal surgery. The rate has risen from 3–4 percent to between 20 percent and 25 percent currently, with figures highest in the Northeast, and lowest, but also rising, in the Midwest. In some hospitals it is 30 percent. In Europe also the Cesarean rate is rising, but the original Cesarean rate there was lower than that of the United States.

The fear of unnecessary Cesareans, and the knowledge that even some of the necessary ones are the ultimate result of routine obstetrical interventions, has confirmed the view that hospital birth is risky and has helped to spark the trend toward midwife birth and home birth.

Childbirth education associations across the country have enlarged the scope of their activity to include consideration of Cesarean birth. Before the increased Cesarean rate these organizations sponsored instruction only in normal childbirth and natural childbirth methods. Political activity was directed toward making possible natural childbirth and family-centered care, including breast-feeding. Medicine was left to the physician. However, these organizations have become involved in the Cesarean question because so many normal women are having Cesareans. As we saw earlier, routine hospital procedures, used for normal women, have the potential to lead to a Cesarean birth.

In 1963 the ratio of live births to obstetricians was 261–1. By 1975 the ratio was 145–1. Nevertheless, the income of obstetricians, with only modest increases in fees, rose dramatically, surpassing even that of general surgeons to make it the highest paid specialty. Cesareans, costing three times as much as a normal delivery, are assumed to be the reason. This writer does not suggest that more Cesareans are being done solely for monetary reasons. Rather, many obstetricians tend to feel that Cesareans are a safe and predictable method of birth.

## THE CESAREAN SURGERY

In a Cesarean, the baby is delivered through the uterine and abdominal walls. Cesareans may be elective, meaning planned ahead of time, and they can be done either before or after labor begins.

The types of Cesarean surgery differ by the location and direction of the uterine incision. The abdominal incision will be vertical and several inches in length from below the navel to just above the pubic hair line. Or it may be the "bikini" incision, somewhat more difficult to do. The second incision, the uterine incision, may be one of three types. It may be made vertically (the classic incision) above the lower part of the uterus, and this is the type used most commonly for emergencies because it can be done fast and can be extended in length if necessary. Or a low vertical incision may be made. The other type is the low cervical incision which is made crosswise in the lower part of the uterus. With this type of incision, there is easier repair of tissue, less bleeding, and more complete healing. It also allows the possibility of a vaginal delivery for a subsequent birth. Most uterine incisions are the low cervical type. If the other type is done, the obstetrician should have good reason.

For Cesarean surgery, the woman is placed on the operating table. She is completely draped except for her face and a small area where the abdominal incision will be made. A screen at chest level prevents her in most cases from seeing the surgery. Sometimes women object to the screen. They feel disembodied. Some wish to see their babies lifted out. If a woman doesn't want a screen, this must be arranged for in advance, probably with the anesthesiology department.

Usually, both arms are strapped at right angles to the sides, with an IV for fluids attached to one arm. Sometimes arrangements can be made to have only that arm, not both, strapped down.

The baby is usually out within a few minutes. The remainder of the time on the table is spent suturing first the uterus, then other layers of tissue including the abdomen. A hundred years ago only the abdomen was stitched, not the uterus. As a result, only the infant lived. Stainless steel surgical staples instead of stitches may be used for the abdominal skin. Sometimes the uterus is lifted out and placed on the abdomen for easier suturing. The father and the mother, too, if she is awake has a free hand, can touch and hold the baby while the obstetrician is closing the incision.

Increasingly, fathers are welcome at Cesarean births. Fathers may talk to their wives or stand up to watch the baby emerge from the slit in the green sheets over the wife's abdomen.

Films of Cesarean birth are available for parents anticipating this type of delivery. Hospital or consumer-oriented Cesarean birth classes may be available. Parents should touch base with them as part of their preparation for the birth.

## ANESTHESIA FOR CESAREANS

The anesthesia, described in Chapter Four, may be regional, that is, a spinal or epidural, or it may be general, which renders the woman unconscious. Most women prefer regional anesthesia, which allows them to be awake for the birth. Regional anesthesia is also safer for both the mother and the baby.

In some hospitals, fathers are allowed only if the mother is awake, the reasoning being that he is there to support her and inform her of what is happening in case the baby is out of her view. However, other hospitals allow the father to be present for the Cesarean even if the mother is asleep. In this case, the reasoning is that since she must miss the birth, he, at least, will be there to take pictures of the baby or describe the birth to her later.

Although the risks of anesthesia are minimal, the couple should be informed and in most cases have a say in the final decision about anesthesia. A need for a sudden Cesarean may indicate general anesthesia, which can be administered faster than regional. Certain back problems may contraindicate spinal anesthesia. Many parents prefer the epidural anyway, because the anesthetic is more controllable, does not enter the spinal fluid, and allows for faster recovery. Also, chills often follow a spinal, and a spinal headache is not uncommon. With an epidural, or even at times a spinal, there may be a feeling of tugging as the baby is lifted out. While some women may be frightened by this, others enjoy the feeling of knowing that their baby is exiting their body. "I couldn't participate in the birth, but I felt more as if I had had a birth when I felt the baby lifted out," one woman told me.

If general anesthesia is required or preferred, it does pass to the baby, although the baby is delivered very soon after it is given. With general anesthesia the baby may be less alert. Also, an endotracheal tube is placed in the mother's throat, and the anesthesiologist controls her breathing by mechanical means because her muscles of respiration have been temporarily paralyzed. With general anesthesia there is, of course, loss of opportunity for immediate bonding with the baby.

If they have had regional anesthesia, women who have had Cesareans can right after birth bond with their baby and even nurse the baby. Later on, when the anesthesia wears off, they will feel pain, so there is an advantage to enjoying the baby while the anesthesia is still effective.

Premedication and postoperative medication must be discussed with the obstetrician. Many women refuse the preop medication designed to calm them before surgery because it will make them less alert after the birth. And they also usually prefer to use minimal pain medication afterward because it passes to the baby through the milk. There are other ways of helping to relieve discomfort. Many women prefer to lie on their sides. After the operation, breathing exercises help clear the lungs of mucus from the anesthesia. After the surgery women can walk within a few hours, usually, but may hold onto their stomachs to support sore muscles.

## AFTER THE CESAREAN

The staples or stitches in the abdomen may be removed in about four days by the obstetrician.

During the surgery the bladder is moved out of the way of the uterus (the tissue must be separated surgically) and then returned to its original position. The catheter, put in place to collect urine at the time of the surgery, is usually left in place for the first couple of days afterward.

An IV is in place for a couple of days after delivery. The woman is not allowed to eat because of "gassiness" following the operation. During surgery, the handling of the intestines in the opened abdomen contributes to this symptom. After a couple of days, Jell-O, and clear liquids, soft food, and finally a regular hospital diet is allowed. Some women find it more difficult to produce milk with this regimen. Many women want the IV removed sooner than two days. Some say they wish to eat regardless of the gassiness, since the discomfort is not very much increased. They find the combination of fasting during labor and after the operation too stressful for their bodies. Besides trying to make milk, their bodies have a major healing process to undertake.

# RISKS OF CESAREAN DELIVERY
# TO WOMAN AND BABY

The availability of "safe" Cesareans is one reason for their increased use. The problems appear to be few. Antibiotics and blood transfusions are readily available, as is resuscitative equipment for the woman and baby. Therefore, this surgery is no longer a matter of last resort to be used only when the woman is already in serious difficulty. It can also be used preventively, or "prophylactically." Cesareans have largely replaced breech delivery and deliveries requiring mid-forceps when the baby is high in the birth canal.

## Complications of Cesarean Delivery
## for the Mother

Just because Cesareans can be done relatively safely is not a reason to perceive them as hardly more than "abdominal birth," as opposed to vaginal birth.

The maternal mortality for Cesareans is 1 in 1,000 births, or four times that of vaginal birth. Half of the increased risk is due to the risks of surgery. The other half is due to the conditions requiring the surgery. (Some dispute these figures, claiming the risk to be twenty-six times that of vaginal birth.)

Almost all women have postoperative pain and gas, as described before. Most still have future Cesareans for delivery, although this is changing (see "Medical Indications for Cesareans," below).

Intrauterine infection rates are 35–65 percent if internally monitored, and 20–40 percent if no monitor is used. Childbed fever is not eliminated. Thus, a rise in temperature postpartum requires attention, even if it is only the flu. However, there is no reason for a mother to be separated from her baby because of a fever. Some elevated temperatures may be simply the result of the stress of surgery.

More rarely, there is the possibility of hemorrhage, adhesions, problems with the incision, injury to adjacent structures such as the ureter and bladder, and complications associated with blood transfusions. Still more rare, but possible, are problems from blood clots, including clots in the lungs, and anesthesia accidents. There is a ½–2 percent chance of subsequent uterine rupture in a future pregnancy. Seventy percent of these ruptures occur before labor begins.

To summarize, the woman after Cesarean surgery will feel intestinal and abdominal pain, perhaps also nausea. She may get a spinal headache. She may get severe chills and shaking after the surgery because of the lowered blood pressure from the spinal and the fact that the blood flows to the surface of the body. In addition, the cold operating room, the removal of the paper or cloth drapes, the thin hospital gown now pulled over her hips, delays in getting blankets, and altered body chemistry for many hours of labor may all contribute to the problem. She can also get an infection from the catheterization procedure.

Feelings generally range from disappointment to depression after a Cesarean. A sense of being deprived is almost universal. Because parents feel fortunate in getting a healthy baby and must deal with the physical concerns of postoperative care, these feelings may not be expressed. Women may feel guilty about acknowledging them even to themselves. They will always have a long scar from below the navel to the top of the pubic hair, although its color will fade. They seldom comment on this as a legitimate complaint. If the Cesarean may have been unnecessary (because a lively, pink, healthy baby emerged with no sign of the fetal distress that was the ostensible reason for the surgery), the parents may prefer not to think about it. They defend their Cesarean experience as nevertheless a birth. They want the birth day to be one of joy, despite the surgery. Later, when there is time to think, some parents may become angry.

## Complications of Cesarean Birth for the Infant

Low birth weight can be a problem since Cesareans may be performed too early despite diagnostic ultrasound and other tests for lung function. Jaundice is the most frequent complication. Respiratory distress follows close behind. Both of these are at least partly associated with low birth weight, although respiratory distress is generally more common with Cesarean babies than those who have experienced the chest compression and labor contractions of vaginal birth, factors which are considered an aid to breathing. There are also drug effects from regional or general anesthesia and from preoperative medications.

How serious these effects are depends on the degree. Babies may be sent to special-care nurseries or neonatal intensive-care units where they may receive oxygen and be monitored in various ways. Their blood will be checked. They may be partly or entirely tube fed at first, although mothers may touch and hold them, and breast-feeding is usually encouraged by hospital staff.

Some parents prefer to plan ahead for the time and date of the Cesarean so that the operating team can be gathered. Others, although anticipating Cesarean, prefer to go into labor spontaneously before the surgery for two reasons. The first is that this way there seem to be fewer respiratory problems after the birth, perhaps because of the gentle stimulation of the contractions. The second is that there is less chance of producing a premature baby. The ultrasound picture can give an indication, although two-dimensional, of infant size, but it is less accurate in the latter part of pregnancy. An amniocentesis can be performed to ascertain lung maturity, but even so, there are more respiratory problems, probably because the infant's lungs are not cleared by being squeezed through the birth canal. After the birth, some parents want input into the number of possible lung X rays that may be given the baby with breathing problems, because of concern about radiation exposure.

Cesarean babies are likely to be sent to a special-care nursery either as a preventive measure or because of a perceived respiratory difficulty. The new parents may question whether or not the separation from the baby at this important time is necessary or desirable. If the husband follows the infant into the nursery, he must then leave his wife who is recovering from the anesthesia.

## Factors Contributing to the Increased Cesarean Rate

A U. S. Government report in 1980 lists the threat of malpractice suits as the most significant factor. Obstetrical policy of a repeat Cesarean section after a previous one is second in importance. Obstetrical training is third (because obstetricians are no longer trained to perform breech birth and are encouraged to do Cesareans in many instances). Belief in superior outcome from Cesarean sections was listed as fourth, followed by changing and expanded indications for Cesarean section.

Age, fertility characteristics, economic class, obstetrical technology, and birth weight were, in descending order, the next-most important factors, followed by severe medical conditions (such as diabetes and herpes infection). All of these factors are discussed in the following pages.

Factors influencing whether a birth will be by Cesarean are described by an International Childbirth Education Association publication. They are ranked from most important to least important:

1. Choice of practitioner and birth location
2. Induction of labor
3. Early intervention in normal labor
4. Maternal position during labor
5. Electronic fetal monitoring
6. Epidural anesthesia
7. Analgesia and sedatives

These factors have been discussed in depth in Chapters Three and Four.

## PREVENTING CESAREANS

The ICEA emphasizes the importance of comprehensive childbirth education courses. To help prevent Cesareans, couples should learn self-help activities such as constant emotional support, position changes, walking during labor, and breathing and relaxation techniques. Drugs and procedures not medically essential should be avoided. Obstetrical procedures and their relationship to possible Cesareans should be learned before delivery. Personal and medical choices during pregnancy and labor that may enhance the likelihood of vaginal birth should be included in childbirth classes. Indications for a Cesarean should be discussed in classes, and information should be given on the advantages of going into labor spontaneously and having a trial labor before a Cesarean is performed.

It is vital for a couple to remember that what happens in labor (and pregnancy) may influence whether or not a Cesarean birth occurs. Couples do have an impact on what happens, even though obstetrician attitudes have moved toward greater reliance on Cesarean birth.

To date there has been no legal action brought for an unnecessary Cesarean, although suits have been brought for not performing a needed one. Therefore, the physician feels more protected doing a Cesarean—and also is rewarded in money and in time saved. Suits involving Cesareans have been brought, however, related to events that occurred during the surgery.

Obstetricians have long been criticized for their lack of training for normal birth and preventative health education. There is the concern currently that in many ways they are not trained for complicated childbirth, either. This includes a lack of education in sexuality, nutrition, exercise, lactation, the psychology of birth, comfort techniques for labor, and non-surgical delivery, without an episiotomy. Consumer groups have urged that physicians-in-training sit with and work with couples through at least one entire labor, as do nursing students and midwives. However, they are trained for pathology, and theirs is still a surgical specialty. If any part of the baby other than the head is first, if the labor is long or the fetal heart changes its rate, if the mother is diabetic or her blood pressure goes up, the solution is likely to be a Cesarean.

David Stewart, executive director of the National Association of Parents and Professionals for Safe Alternatives in Childbirth, describes the five standards for safe childbirth. They are good nutrition, skillful midwifery, natural childbirth, birth at home, and breast-feeding.

There are indeed factors in hospitals that contribute to otherwise unnecessary Cesareans. Many relate to the routine obstetrical interventions described in Chapter Four. When this is pointed out to obstetricians, some say, "Nothing is routine in medicine. We only use them when we have to. Most women need them." Others say, "We do the routine procedures 'prophylactically,' as a preventive measure."

Cesareans have become so accepted among many obstetricians that they are hardly seen as a complication. Many obstetricians believe that they are indeed the safest solution for birth. Refusal of a Cesarean has even been claimed to constitute child abuse. If a woman has a sick baby and refused permission for surgery, she should, says a spokesman of the American College of Obstetrics and Gynecology, be held liable. He does not mention, however, the infant deaths as a result of Cesareans nor infant illness from respiratory disease and low birth weight.

## MEDICAL INDICATIONS FOR CESAREANS

Sometimes Cesarean surgery must be done, and it can indeed be lifesaving. Here are some possible medical reasons for the surgery:

a) *CPD,* or cephalopelvic disproportion, where the baby's head appears too large to fit through the pelvis or is extended with the chin out rather than flexed toward the chest. Midwives have always had special training to ascertain the architecture of the pelvis and to assess the size and position of the baby without the use of ultrasound. CPD is a possibility if the baby has not "dropped" before labor or does not drop during early labor. Possibly there is a lack of pelvic space.

A chief obstetrician, in a newspaper interview, stated that the increased number of Cesareans are done as a result of babies' heads getting larger because of better nutrition, and that women's pelvises had not increased to compensate! Actually, babies' average weights during the past twenty years have increased by no more than two ounces.

Possible CPD is given as a reason for using ultrasound several times during pregnancy, even with no assurance of the procedure's long-term safety. Is the baby "large for dates"? Although only two-dimensional, ultrasound pictures help to determine whether the baby is large enough for induced labor or Cesarean, or is getting too large and therefore should be induced or delivered by section. Many women insist on a trial of labor regardless of ultrasound results. A large baby is not more difficult to deliver than a small baby provided that the head fits through the pelvis.

Is there IUGR (intrauterine growth retardation)? Babies with small heads may also be delivered by Cesarean for fear that they are small because of inadequate placental function. There is a desire to get them out of the women and into the perceived safety of the intensive-care nursery.

Labor is usually allowed to progress in the case of CPD, because diagnosis of the condition is not a science, but an educated guess. If the woman is undrugged, walks, squats down on her heels, and keeps her bladder empty, there may be adequate space for a vaginal birth. If she lies on her back with epidural anesthesia during labor, she may well have a Cesarean.

**b)** *Uterine Dystocia,* or "lazy uterus." No one knows how long labor should be or exactly what is "abnormal labor pattern." Because it takes nine hours to get to 3–4 centimeters of cervical dilation does not mean the labor will be eighteen to twenty hours. The cervix dilates at an ever-increasing rate, and the last 2–3 centimeters of dilation occur usually in less than an hour.

One woman says, "My labor was an off-again-on-again labor for four days. The Braxton-Hicks contractions gradually turned into a labor of sorts on Monday. The baby and I were fine. I ate, napped, even walked around the neighborhood. I delivered on Friday at home. No sweat. In the hospital I would have been sectioned for sure. The baby was in a slightly posterior position, but when she suddenly turned anterior she came fast. It was a great birth."

The use of Pitocin to speed the contractions of a "lazy" uterus may result in a slowed fetal heartbeat—and a consequent section. On the other hand, if no Pitocin is used and the labor does not progress fast enough, a section will also be done. The hosptial is not organized to hold couples for an extended time before the birth.

An "older woman"—sometimes meaning even as young as thirty—may be given less time to labor. Older women are variously assumed to have fast labors, especially if they have had previous children, or slow labors because the uterus is assumed to be "lazy" and the tissues non-elastic. There is no evidence for either assumption.

Maternal stress may slow labor. One woman relates, "I was the labor support for a friend. They got her into the hospital early before she'd had any sleep that night, because her waters had broken. They kept her up all night, monitored her, fed her nothing, kept worrying her about progress and a possible section. No wonder the woman couldn't do her labor. I wish I could have taken her home to let her rest and eat. But, of course, she was sectioned for 'failure to progress'."

"Failure to Progress," another term for uterine dystocia, is the most common reason for Cesareans. Unrealistic expectations about the length of labor abound. Normal labor has become defined not as fourteen to eighteen hours for a first baby, but as short as ten or even eight hours. As couples are entering the hospital later in labor, obstetrical staff become accustomed to all deliveries occurring within a few hours of admission. The pressure to accept monitoring, Pitocin, and ultimately a Cesarean can be described frequently as assaultive, even though hospital staff truly believe that the mother is fatigued and the baby in jeopardy. An occasional obstetrician will admit, "It's hard after a long day to wait around an extra few hours in case she progresses when you know she may need a section anyway." It is a dilemma.

c) *Premature Rupture of Membranes.* This might also be placed in the category of "failure to progress." If ruptured membranes are the first sign of labor, or if they are ruptured by hospital staff to speed labor or to insert an electrode for the fetal heart monitor, an artificial time limit is placed on labor because of the possibility of infection.

The woman in labor must accept Pitocin or move ahead quickly on her own to avoid the "failure to progress" Cesarean. She may be "allowed" forty-eight hours, but it may be as short as twenty-four hours, even with no internal exams or internal monitor.

Some women may try to sleep and avoid reporting the water breaking to gain more time. An obstetrician says, "I agree with that. Especially if they break at night, she should stay home and sleep. If she comes in, the staff wonder why I don't 'Pit' her [give Pitocin] or section her by afternoon." The relationship between length of labor, use of Pitocin, and breaking of membranes (whether spontaneously or artificially), was discussed in detail in Chapter Four.

d) *Previous Cesarean Section.* "Once a C-section, always a C-section" was pronounced with its rhythmic cadence for sixty-four years. Physicians have been genuinely concerned about allowing a vaginal birth after a Cesarean. They are not reassured that scar tissue is strong, although no such fears have been expressed about episiotomy scar tissue. Although ½ to 2 percent of previous Cesarean incisions may rupture, because 70 percent of these occur before delivery, the number of ruptures during labor is small.

C-Sec, Inc. (66 Christopher Road, Waltham, MA 02154) has been the prime force in educating women about Cesareans, the indications for them, how to avoid them, and how to have optimal Cesarean experience. This organization, not satisfied with the dictum, "Once a Cesarean, always a Cesarean" has also pressed for information about vaginal birth after Cesarean birth. One of the original founders of C-Sec had a vaginal birth after a Cesarean, and then a third vaginal birth at home. She has founded a new organization with classes for couples planning a vaginal birth after a Cesarean delivery. It's called Vaginal Birth After Cesarean (VBAC), and is located at 118 Great Plain Terrace in Needham, Massachusetts, under the leadership of Nancy Cohen.

There has been, until recent public pressure was exerted, little incentive for obstetricians to allow a normal birth after a Cesarean. If the mother comes in early, as she will in this situation, they may have to spend a great deal of time with her. There is a strong incentive to do the section early, electively, at a planned time without even a trial of labor. ("What's the point in exhausting her for nothing when the labor may not work anyway?" even though a trial of labor is preferred by most informed parents.)

How long the trial labor should continue depends on circumstances. The mother may need a Cesarean after all. If there are any problems, the obstetrician feels liable if he does not perform the surgery. The woman may not be comfortable with the idea of vaginal birth or willing to confront the fact that her first Cesarean may not have been necessary. The Cesarean will cost in total three times that of vaginal birth, but that is of little concern to the patient because the patient seldom pays the fee.

A Bronx, New York, hospital study results of vaginal birth after Cesarean showed that of 65 percent of women with previous sections delivered vaginally. Also in New York City, an Albert Einstein Hospital study showed a 51 percent success rate. Excluded from both studies were women who had had more than one previous section or who had a contracted pelvis or chronic disease. Generally, the repeat section rate, which used to be 98 percent, has begun to drop as a result of public pressure and a recent year-long federal government study by an appointed Task Force.

Women have questioned their obstetricians about the need for a Cesarean birth, and have usually been intimidated with a response indicating that their desires for a vaginal birth are selfish and self-indulgent, a frill, even. Their baby's safety, it is claimed, requires the sacrifice. This is often said with a matter-of-factness that seems incredible considering the years of infant exposure to drugs and forceps to the point of requiring resuscitation for normal newborns. The desire for spontaneous, undrugged vaginal birth, too, was once greeted as a self-indulgence that could be dispensed with. Physicians may prefer to see birth as a series of medical events, not as a quite normal biological function.

The 1980 Task Force on Cesarean Section convened by the National Institute of Child Health and Human Development in Washington, D.C., stated after a year's study that the dramatic upsurge in the rate of Cesarean births in the United States could be halted and perhaps reversed without harm to infants or mothers. The seventeen members included twelve physicians, a medical statistician, a psychologist, an economist, a medical sociologist, a lawyer, and just one consumer, the well-known Elizabeth Shearer, who has studied Cesarean birth extensively.

Public testimony was severely limited, though parents who had been harmed or had had their children harmed by Cesarean section sought to present evidence.

The Task Force suggested that physicians scrutinize the reason for first Cesareans and consider non-surgical methods such as allowing a woman in labor to rest, walk around, and drink fluids in an attempt to achieve a normal vaginal birth.

Repeat sections account for 27 percent of the total rise in the Cesarean rate since 1970. Without a change in the repeat Cesarean policy, the total Cesarean rate will continue to rise. The Task Force suggested modifying the old dictum about repeat sections.

The panel decided that the labor trial should take place in a hospital with staff available to perform an emergency Cesarean if necessary. The previous incision should have been a low uterine "bikini" incision, they stated.

Women are now often able to find a physician who will allow a vaginal delivery after a Cesarean. The major complaint is that the trial of labor is too short, and that the Cesarean is done within a few hours of admission before labor is really under way because the parents come, in this case, to the hospital very early in the labor usually at the obstetrician's request.

The Task Force defined physician fears of malpractice and failure to progress as the major factors in the primary section rate. Physicians' claims of delivering "better babies" through Cesareans could not be documented.

Helen Marieskind, Doctor of Public Health, was contracted by HEW to evaluate the Cesarean rate. Her report, completed in 1979 and released in 1980, states that half the repeat sections could have been avoided at a saving of $95 million. She also stated that there is no evidence showing that increased Cesarean rate is producing healthier babies.

e) *Breech Birth.* Already alluded to, babies in the breech position constitute 3.5 percent of all births. Many are initially breeched, but then assume a head-down position before the last weeks of pregnancy. Some are not diagnosed as breech babies until labor. The fear is that the cord may get compressed, or that the head, larger than the body, may not fit through the pelvis after delivery of the body. Skill and constant assessment of the baby can minimize this risk. Sometimes obstetricians are successful in turning a breech into a vertex, or head-down position.

The Task Force on Cesarean Section has suggested that a breech baby weighing under eight pounds with normal pelvic structure could be delivered vaginally if the physician is experienced in vaginal birth.

f) *Other Indications* for a Cesarean might be the appearance of meconium from the baby's intestines combined with a lowered fetal heart rate (of 100–115, for example). True maternal exhaustion or hypertension not explained by the birth environment could also be an indication. Diabetes is still a frequent indication because diabetic women tend to delay going into labor, and sugar metabolism for mother and baby must be monitored. True post-maturity, for example, three weeks beyond the expected date, combined with tests for placental function may indicate the need for an induced labor. A failed induction will require a Cesarean.

Genital herpes, a sexually transmitted disease on the rise, has no known cure. If the virus is active at the time of delivery, the baby can get infected as it passes through the vagina. Therefore, a Cesarean must be done.

Toxemia of pregnancy, as discussed earlier under possible complications in Chapter One, will likely require a Cesarean delivery. Induction of labor may be tried first.

A transverse baby, i.e., where the baby lies across the uterus, requires a Cesarean.

Twins are now often considered a reason for a Cesarean, because the second may be in the breech position. Also, labor may be longer with twins. Having been taken surgically, the twins may be held in the intensive-care unit, but the outcome appears more certain. The obstetrician wants to see immediately that both twins are healthy without waiting for labor. There is, however, some controversy on this point. Formerly, of course, twins were usually born vaginally. Anyone expecting a multiple birth should read Elizabeth Noble's, *Having Twins*.

Previous extensive uterine surgery, as for fibroids, may require a Cesarean.

A February 1982 article in the *New England Journal of Medicine* gave some evidence of increased safety of Cesareans for low-birth-weight babies, but many variables were not considered. The mortality for infants, as opposed to fetal death, was not reduced. Morbidity was not studied. Forceps use was not recorded, only that surgery produced a live baby. The study acknowledged that a stillbirth was more likely to be delivered vaginally to spare the mother unnecessary surgery, and it was noted that this could improve the figures for Cesarean sections.

## Emergency Cesareans

If the head is engaged in the pelvis prior to labor, there is no reason to be concerned about *cord prolapse* (where the cord comes first and is therefore in danger of being compressed). In the case of compression, an emergency Cesarean may be done, or the woman may get into the knee-chest position and be able to deliver her baby vaginally. Sometimes forceps are used to hasten delivery.

*Premature separation of the placenta* is usually a reason for an emergency Cesarean unless the separation is only partial and birth is imminent. No one knows why this problem occurs. It may result from pressure applied on the abdomen to speed the second stage. Poor prenatal nutrition could be a factor, although it is difficult to study this cause-and-effect relationship.

If the placenta is over the cervix blocking the baby's descent, a Cesarean is also required. This may not be an emergency, however. It is known perhaps because the head remains high, and it is diagnosed by ultrasound.

## OBSTETRICAL INTERVENTION AND CESAREANS

A hospital childbirth educator reports that she and her assistant have remarkable success in predicting which four women in the class of sixteen apparently normal mothers-to-be will have a C-section. "They usually appear passive. They trust their doctors and feel disloyal in doubting or questioning the doctor's judgment. They are pleased when their doctor compliments them for gaining only two or three pounds. They are upset if he criticizes them for gaining. They expect to be taken care of. Our talk of patient rights and the importance of communication doesn't elicit any real response. They appear puzzled sometimes. People who wish to avoid a Cesarean have to take good care of themselves and take knowledgeable responsibility. Those who don't risk being 'finished up' so their doctor can get home."

In summary:

Going to the hospital too early can lead to a C-section.

Rupturing the membranes to speed labor can lead to a C-section.

An IV can lead to a C-section, whether or not it contains Pitocin.

The use of Pitocin to stimulate or "improve" labor can lead to a C-section.

Staying in bed, especially on one's back during labor can lead to a C-section.

Expressing anxiety "to get it over with" or complaining of fatigue can lead to a C-section.

Prolonged fasting during labor can lead to fatigue and a C-section.

The use of a fetal heart monitor of whatever type can lead to a C-section.

A full bladder can lead to a C-section.

An intermittent, on-again-off-again labor can lead to a C-section.

Comments about lack of progress by obstetrical staff can tip the scales toward a C-section.

Epidural anesthesia can lead to a C-section.

A Cesarean section may be truly necessary, and a Cesarean birth can be a joyful birth. However, choices made during labor, which could lead to an otherwise unnecessary Cesarean, need to be considered.

# Chapter Eight

# HOME BIRTH, ALTERNATIVE BIRTH CENTERS, AND MIDWIVES

Home birth, birth in homelike alternative birth centers, and midwife attendance at birth are recent options for parents-to-be.

Some in the health-care delivery system expect—even hope—that these options may be fads that will one day go away. At an earlier time natural childbirth and family-centered hospital care were often perceived as different from mainstream obstetrics, demanded by a persistent few, and unavailable to most. At times, natural childbirth, rooming-in, and husband participation in birth were seen less as innovative than fanatical; and it was believed that if professional lines held firm against public pressure, and the banner of safety was waved with enough vigor, these requests would go away.

Couples who choose out-of-hospital birth uniformly find it a satisfying, fulfilling experience. They tell their friends. They may invite their friends. That it is merely a fad seems unlikely.

## HOME BIRTH

Home birth first became an option in the mid-seventies. A very few people had made arrangements to deliver at home before that time, but by the mid-seventies there were planned programs across the country.

Organized groups educated their instructors and began sponsoring classes, which have developed along lines similar to those of the childbirth education organizations. These associations may even offer a home-birth class in addition to preparing couples for hospital birth. Of course, there is no planned program of hospital staff education as there is for prepared childbirth. Instead, arrangements are made with hospitals for backup care. Some medical and nursing students, also staff members, are curious about the why and the how of home birth. However, their contacts with classes and attendance at a home birth may be surreptitious because the medical establishment generally opposes home birth.

The executive director of the American College of Obstetrics and Gynecology expressed his views in a 1980 issue of the "College Newsletter": "One of the health-care issues most frustrating to Fellows has been home birth. Physician concerns for the well-being of both mother and newborn seem not to be shared by some pregnant couples who speak of 'experiences' instead of outcomes."

There are physicians, nurses, and other health professionals who support responsible home birth, though. There is even a small physician organization for home birth, the American College of Home Obstetrics.

The International Childbirth Education Association supports home birth, but with guidelines. These include attendance by certified midwives or physicians in consultation with obstetric and pediatric specialists, backup care, prenatal care, screening for high-risk women, a prior home visit, home preparation with adequate supplies and transportation, and newborn examination, and follow-up.

## Why Home Birth?

Basically, for those who choose home birth, the original reasons for going to the hospital no longer exist, except when specific hospital services are required. Pain is no longer the overriding issue that shapes the entire experience of childbirth. Couples no longer believe that hospitals are cleaner with fewer disease-causing organisms than homes. They no longer believe that for normal birth the hospital is the safest place to be. They learn about birth and how to use the hospital.

The difficulties of avoiding routine hospital interventions, including Cesareans, and the desire to avoid unpleasantness during labor and delivery are major reasons for the surge in home births. Parents see the risks in hospitals. The statement is frequently heard that, "Anyone who wants a normal birth will have to stay home." It is not the homemade quilts or the plants that keep couples home, as some have suggested. They also enjoy the autonomy and intimacy of home birth and the continuing supportive care and consultation that replace the hospital's intermittent, authoritarian directives, that sometimes treat the parents themselves as children.

Here are some parents' comments:

"If we have an unavoidable, unhappy experience, we want it to be at least our own experience. We don't want to live with a nothing experience or a mucked-up hospital experience."

"We like the home-birth classes. We can focus on birth instead of spending energy wondering how to cope with the hospital or obstetrician. At our last birth in the hospital we felt verbally assaulted even though we got what we wanted. I delivered in what looked like an ICU [intensive-care unit]."

"Whatever happened to our plans for natural childbirth? We got in there [the hospital] and all sorts of things happened which we didn't expect. Nothing we said seemed to make any difference. I didn't want my vagina cut for delivery. The nurses said, 'You should have gotten that from your classes.'"

Lester Hazell, a former president of the International Childbirth Education Association and a member of the faculty of the School of Nurse-Midwifery at the University of California in San Diego, did a study in the mid-seventies of 300 elective home births on the West Coast. Results showed that couples who chose home birth were above average in socioeconomic and educational status and sense of responsibility for their families.

## How Safe is Home Birth?

Most people over age sixty today were born at home. Home birth was popular longer in Europe than in America. In Holland the majority of babies are still born at home, with midwives in attendance, although political forces there are acting to move birth to hospitals. Holland has long had the lowest infant death rate of any developed country, while the United States, where hospital birth is the rule, has had one of the highest infant-mortality rates.

Infant mortality has been steadily declining for a hundred years regardless of the place of birth. Safe surgery, antibiotics, better living conditions, communicable disease control and treatment, and public health laws protecting contamination of food, water, and milk have all contributed to the decline.

Home birth today has improved from the home-birth experience earlier in this century. There is now knowledge of birth processes, prenatal exercise, and comfort techniques for labor. The "what ifs" are knowable and generally treatable. Medical tools and expertise are quickly available.

Interestingly, the safety of the earlier home-birth services to poor women has never been equaled in hospital birth. The famed Frontier Nursing Service in Kentucky, in the days before it had its own hospital, delivered poorly nourished women with many children in their mountain homes. Yet the death rate for both women and babies was less than the United States average at that time. Their figures are at least as good as current U.S. statistics, and many feel that the safety exceeded that of normal hospital birth even today. For twenty-three years there was not a single maternal death. The Chicago Maternity Center had 12,000 births without a single maternal death at a time when the United States rate was two per thousand. The New York Maternity Center Association had a similarly extraordinary safety record. These midwifery services had no medical supervision and no backup facilities.

The medical schools continued to offer home-birth services until the 1940s, but few ever even investigated the home before delivery to ascertain suitability for a birth. The doctors, who were usually students, were inadequately trained. Members of the family sometimes gave chloroform if needed for pain relief. Yet the home-delivery service of the former Boston Lying-In Hospital had safety figures better than those of any of the hospitals. In fact, in hospitals it was noted that between 1918 and 1925 infant deaths from birth injuries rose 5 percent each year. In 1933 a White House Conference revealed that maternal mortality had not declined between 1915 and 1930, the years during which birth moved to the hospital.

Neal Devitt, M.D., a resident in Family Practice at the University of California performed a study on home birth. His conclusion was:

> While the techniques of modern hospital obstetrics have saved the lives of many women and infants from genuine pathologies of birth, the literature of obstetrics in the United States from 1930 to 1960 does not show that healthy women with normal pregnancies benefitted from hospital obstetric care. Although statistically inconclusive, most of the studies done of home and hospital birth from this period shows that the incidence of birth injuries and obstetric mortality was greater in hospitals, probably due to interference in the birth process. These studies suggest that despite the poverty, ill health and frequent high-risk conditions of women who delivered at home, and despite the frequent poor training of attendants, and anesthesia used—often in crowded, unsanitary settings—home birth was not less safe than hospital birth from 1930 to 1960.

Studies by home-birth organizations, university researchers, and others are being done of modern home birth with healthy women, trained in childbirth, with experienced attendants, and with medical backup. The safety is uniformly good.

Lewis Mehl, M.D., formerly at the University of Wisconsin Medical School, studied two matched groups of over 1,000 newborns in Madison, Wisconsin. Hospital births had six times the fetal distress of home birth, four times as much infant resuscitation and infection, three times the number of Cesarean sections, nine times the number of episiotomies and tears, and thirty times more birth injuries. Birth injuries, most of which were associated with forceps, included cephalohematomas (bruise on head) and resulting jaundice, facial nerve paralysis, other nerve injuries, broken bones, and fractured skull. These were injuries evident during the first three days of life as recorded in hospital charts. Later problems and long-term effects, therefore, were not included in the study.

Clearly, long-held assumptions about hospital safety are undergoing reconsideration.

## Who Delivers the Baby at Home?

Planned home birth is not characterized by a do-it-yourself philosophy. The people who may offer their services for a home delivery are physicians or lay midwives. The physician need not be an obstetrician, although in hospitals general-practice physicians have gradually lost their privileges for delivering babies as the specialty of obstetrics has developed.

Ironically, certified nurse-midwives, on the other hand, in many states have generally lost the privilege of delivering babies at home, but may now deliver in hospitals, where they may even have a physician in the delivery room with them. In other institutions, the midwife delivers, but if a problem arises the obstetrical residents in training are to be called. The nurse-midwife professional organization is the American College of Nurse-Midwives. These midwives are trained both as nurses and as midwives in approved programs. Their privileges vary according to the laws of each state and the regulations developed in hospitals.

Lay midwives may serve as birth attendants. They also deliver babies. Many have circumvented the nursing degree and limited available nurse-midwifery programs to arrange for their own training, of which apprenticeship is an important part. First, as an apprentice, they are present at home births to assist with supplies, prepare food, and care for other children in the home. Later, they learn to take the fetal heart rate and the blood pressures and to perform vaginal exams, and repair vaginal tears. They may keep birth notes, the equivalent of the hospital medical record. They attend home-birth classes and other in-service programs.

Because they do not fall under the regulations of nurse-midwives, they can legally deliver in many states. Some states license them, a few states prohibit them, and in other states their status is unclear.

In a home birth, the parents may catch the baby with the assistance of a physician or lay midwife. Professionals, including nurses, may come as friends without clear-cut roles. Invited friends come to participate in the birth and to help out in ways usually planned long before. Always, hospital backup is an essential part of a planned home birth.

Most physicians avoid home birth and are afraid of it. Professional publications and magazines tell physicians how to deal with patients who present this request. If patients insist, ways are suggested to change their minds. If this fails, physicians are encouraged to be involved in prenatal care, in supervisory roles, and follow-up care. Some physicians refuse to perform prenatal care for couples planning on a home birth in an effort to stamp out the practice. They may state, "I saw a woman go into shock. What if she hadn't been in the hospital?" However, there is no analysis of the prenatal or labor circumstances and medical care in the recounted anecdotes. Home birth may be seen as primitive, as natural childbirth was sometimes described in its early years. Some physicians also fear being ostracized by colleagues.

Pediatricians are frequently available after the birth, and occasionally they come to the home. Most babies are brought to the office after being checked by the home-birth team, either the same day or the next day. Silver nitrate eye drops and vitamin K are not usually used at home births. Circumcision is not common.

Nurse-midwives may or may not be personally supportive of home birth. Many are grateful that they are now accepted into the hospital, even knowing that their acceptance occurs because they draw patients to the institution. Some nurse-midwives are stronger advocates for parents than others.

There exists the possibility, though not common, that the knowledgeable nurse-midwife may "get between" the couple or family members or "take over" the birth. Or if, for example, the midwife has privileges to do episiotomies, she may see them as more necessary than if she is forbidden by law to do the procedure. This concern encourages some families to select lay midwives.

Lay midwives function almost entirely in the home, although they may also accompany women to the hospital for labor support. They are in a less ambiguous position of advocacy and support for consumers.

In the home, whoever the participants, the group is structured to function as a team, without the problems of "turf" that can occur in other settings. All are guests in the home of the parents. They are there because they wish to be. The five-year-old lays out the baby clothes. A friend answers the phone. The midwife team watches, checks. The husband supports and coaches his wife and is in general control of the household. The couple can move about the house if they wish. She can eat and drink. There can be quiet. There can be talk about birth and its progress in which all participate. The couple can find time to be alone if they wish. Or friends may be gathered around. Friends may massage the mother's back and legs. Sometimes they play music if she asks. Some who come will not be in the birth room except for an occasional word of encouragement. Home births are characterized by a sensitivity in human relationships that is almost uncanny.

If the hours of care in home birth were to be financially reimbursed, the expense would be high. Rather, it is a case of women helping women, friends helping friends.

## Preparing for Home Birth

The home does not contain the possibly virulent hospital germs, but home-birth couples should be attentive to cleanliness in the environment. Clean a room, make up the bed for birth, and arrange the supplies so all will be ready, and don't use the room until the birth. If this is not practical, make up the bed at the time of labor. Sheets may be washed with Clorox and soap, ironed or dried in the sun, and wrapped in new plastic bags. Sometimes clothing and bedding are heated in the oven at a low temperature in brown paper bags.

The bed is made first with a plastic sheet or shower curtain against the mattress, then a bed sheet, another plastic sheet and a bed sheet on top. This allows the bed to be changed easily by removing the top layers as blood and leakage of amniotic fluid make the bed wet.

The room should be warmed to about 75° F, which is optimum for the newborn.

Towels and wash cloths are needed, also absorbent disposable pads to place under the woman for leakage of fluid. Sanitary napkins are needed after the birth.

Water is boiled for birth at home, for several purposes. If white shoe strings are used to tie the cord, they will be boiled, as will be the scissors used to cut the cord. Warm, wet compresses to support and relax the vaginal area may be dipped in the still-warm sterile water. Water may also be boiled for tea; perhaps herbal teas.

Disposable cord clamps may be bought at medical-supply houses for about thirty cents. A basin to catch the placenta will also be needed.

Also have on hand an ear syringe, which may be used to suction mucus from the baby's mouth. Babies born at home will seldom need much if any suction, since they will not have been exposed to drugs, forceps, or hospital infections. They will not be premature—the major problem for infants—since if they were, a planned home birth would not have taken place. The doctor or midwife brings a fetascope to listen to the baby's heart during labor, blood pressure equipment, sterile gloves for vaginal exams, and perhaps other supplies depending on backup arrangements. A car filled with gas must be in the driveway in case the couple need to go to the hospital.

Birth attendants come when labor begins, often bringing extra clean clothes and a sleeping bag. They will stay for a time after birth, assisting the father in observing and caring for mother and baby, doing laundry, preparing food, and washing dishes. The father then takes over. One or two friends may stay for a few hours. The grandparents, although usually initially aghast at the idea of not using a hospital, often arrive after the birth, if not before. They tend to become part of the helping team as though they had been doing this for years, and they often express feelings of fulfillment and closeness that they could not have foretold.

## Who Cannot Plan Home Birth

All planned home-birth programs include comprehensive prenatal care, more so than usually found in traditional prenatal visits. Traditional obstetrical care depends on hospitals to treat problems such as prematurity so that obstetrical complications such as anomalies of the pelvic bone structure or infant positions not ideal for delivery can be dealt with later at the birth.

Home-birth organizations usually screen out women who:

1. are under seventeen or, probably, over forty for a first baby
2. are markedly underweight or overweight

3. do not take responsibility for preparing for the birth, or who do not plan to breast feed. They are concerned about women who will not breast feed their newborns, since this runs counter to the philosophy behind a home birth. Also, there are safety considerations, since breast-feeding helps the uterus to contract and ensures that the baby is getting enough nutrients.

4. smoke, drink alcohol, or do not eat a nutritionally adequate prenatal diet

5. have had a previous Cesarean or extensive uterine surgery

6. have an Rh problem

7. are anemic, hypertensive, or diabetic or have cardio-vascular disease

8. have babies in the breech position or not in the usual head-down, chin-flexed position

9. have had more than two miscarriages

10. have a previous history of premature birth

11. have babies more than three weeks before or after the due date

12. have a history of bleeding during pregnancy (other than some staining common in the first two or three months)

13. live more than twenty minutes from a hospital.

See the Appendix for where to write for more information on home birth.

## ALTERNATIVE BIRTH CENTERS

Those who feel comfortable with neither hospital nor home birth may choose an alternative birth center. These centers, usually independent of hospitals, are administered by nurse-midwives with obstetricians available if needed. At least one is operated by an obstetrician.

Included is comprehensive prenatal care, childbirth education, welcoming of the family (including siblings of the new baby), use of a kitchen, extensive father participation, and discharge approximately twelve hours after the birth. Postpartum home visits, or perhaps one or more visits by the couple back to the center are part of the program.

The Maternity Center Association of New York opened the first alternative birth center, accredited in 1979 by the National League of Nursing and the American Public Health Association (APHA). The APHA governing council endorses family-centered childbirth and recognizes the need for options in maternity care. This includes financial resources for out-of-hospital birth such as reimbursement by health insurance companies.

A study of the results of births at out-of-hospital birth centers is being done at eleven centers. There are at least a hundred birth centers now in operation nationwide.

The alternative birth centers are geared to offer truly natural childbirth and family participation. There is no need to defend, for example, the refusal of amniotomies, IVs, monitors, Pitocin, episiotomies, circumcision, vitamin K, and sugar water for babies. There is no need to negotiate bathroom privileges, extra pillows, showers, something to drink, gentle birth, time for nursing and bonding. As a result, the parents are more free to relax, to concentrate on their breathing techniques, and to share the miracle of natural birth.

# Chapter Nine

# PATIENT RIGHTS, PARENT CHOICES

The long-standing admonition, "Trust your doctor," contained the implicit assumption that the consumers of medical services need do no more than comply with the requirements of the medical-care system. Today, this obsolete obeisance to medicine has been superseded by the general recognition that patients have responsibilities that go beyond keeping appointments and accepting treatment. The physician's responsibility has also expanded to include informing patients in order to bring them into the decision-making process. The physician is then in a less vulnerable position if the outcome is unfavorable. For parents and for the child, too, although perhaps less measurably the child, the impact of what happens in childbirth will be long lasting.

No one designed the obstetrical-care system to frustrate parents. In fact, it was not designed at all. It evolved. The obstetrician is accountable for certain aspects of care, but not all of it; nor is the chief of obstetrics, the hospital administrator, the nurses, or the board of trustees. All of these people, and others, too, have a part in it. No ombudsman coordinates the total care of each patient from pregnancy through the various aspects of the hospital experience, through the time immediately following birth, including breast-feeding and early parenting. Family practice medicine, sometimes including both midwifery and home birth among its services, may come close. Lay midwifery services are also able to offer coordinated care for each individual birth experience. But ultimately the responsibility for coordination of care falls to the parents, who are the only persons who experience the sequence of events in their totality. They, accordingly, must learn to select and use services, communicating relevant information. Couples who describe the day of their child's birth as "the most beautiful day of our lives" have usually planned well for that day.

In the 1980 Yale Medical School commencement address the dean, Philip Felig, M.D., stated, "The view of medical practice from outside the profession has taken on negative connotations. The physician more than ever is viewed as a technician eager to apply powerful new methods of diagnosis or treatment, a technician generally indifferent to the patient as a person, unconcerned about the cost to society, and unwilling to share with the patient and society as a whole in the decision-making process."

Many patients will say, "My doctor is not one of those. He knows more than I do. I have faith in him." Many do not wish to acknowledge that everything that happens to them is not done for their benefit. Acknowledging dissatisfaction can be seen as expecting too much or as having erred in selecting the providers of medical care. People are sometimes "grateful for crumbs" from the medical establishment.

Couples often ask what is "allowed" them in the hospital. "Do I have to have a fetal monitor?" They see the doctor and hospital more as giving them permission than as providing consultation and service for them. More parents are asking, "What happens if we refuse something? Do we have the right to refuse obstetrical intervention? Do we talk with our obstetrician about our wishes?"

Obstetricians may say, "I'm tired of hearing about patient rights. What about physicians' rights? I don't have time to explain everything so they can give 'informed consent.' Most of them would only get worried if they heard what could happen." About patient reports of care to childbirth instructors or quotes from parents, they may say, "Those are only anecdotal. There's no proof that what they object to is harmful. Of course, there are some problems. It's risky to cross the street. We're not perfect. We're only human." Sometimes a practice is justified by reference to an article in a professional journal. However, the sample may be only a handful of patients, with no control group and variables ill-defined and unaccounted for. Often, the professional paper also has many elements of the anecdotal. Typical comments are,

"A study shows that home birth is dangerous." And, "We're getting healthier babies with more Cesareans." These are not precise, scientific statements.

Everyone can benefit from reducing the adversary relationship between obstetricians and parents planning natural childbirth. Both favor prepared childbirth and family-centered care. Both see it as having improved the quality of birth. Both have as top priority a healthy baby. However, health is defined as more than the absence of clinical disease, say parents. Health can be a more nebulous concept than that of disease.

As if professional training, institutional needs, and the political impact of the drug and insurance industries weren't enough to divide obstetricians and parents, parents and professionals also have access to different information. Parents may read the professional journals available in medical libraries, but physicians are less likely to read the lay press on health topics and medical care. They did not read them during their training and therefore may not see them as credible. Many of these books for the public attack the medical-care system as not being prevention-oriented, ignoring environmental health concerns, being inadequate in areas of general health, and as "medicalizing" normal life events, such as birth.

Prepared childbirth seems to weaken physicians' authority over the birth process. Many have barely had the opportunity to read even one book on the parents' role in preparing for birth. Until parent pressure became too great to be ignored, a common stance was, "Either you do the birth, or I do it."

Not surprising is the fact that the physician may see prevention in terms of early intervention, or his genuine belief that intervention yields a superior outcome. Therefore, couples may subject the obstetrician to what may seem to him or her an inquisition, while parents hear from their doctor what sounds to them like a patronizing incantation: "It's for your safety." "The hospital requires it." "I only do a procedure when I have to." "We can't take chances." "We're saving babies." "Don't you trust me?" An occasional obstetrician will say, "I intend to give good medical care regardless of parents' desires," thereby not recognizing patient rights or informed consent. These obstetricians will feel more at ease with medicalized childbirth classes taught by the office nurse, than those sponsored by the more consumer-oriented childbirth education organizations. Many obstetricians have no way of relating to the statement by the International Childbirth Education Association that controlling technology is the primary problem in childbirth today. Most do not even know the statement has been made, or, indeed, that the organization even exists.

Couples will not all want the same options for birth. Since most are healthy, there is no medical reason for them to all have the same options. Communication between parents and medical professionals is crucial, and much of the initiative usually must come from parents. A woman who did not achieve this communication reported sadly, "I felt I wasn't invited to my own delivery."

## PLANNING FOR THE BIRTH

There are obstacles to overcome. The first is lack of information about birth, ways of coping with pain, and what to expect in a hospital or out-of-hospital birth.

The second is to recognize that the same questions are being asked of obstetricians nationwide. Individual office encounters can make couples feel that their requests are unusual. They don't know that, in many cases, other patients—even those of the same obstetrician—are thinking or saying the same things.

The third obstacle is the difficulty of evaluating care before the birth. In buying most other services or goods, the guidelines are clearer. In this case, it sometimes seems that the sellers call the tune and tell the customer what they should buy. The consumer's needs are defined by the providers of the services.

The fourth factor with which to deal is the unpredictability of labor patterns, combined with possibly unpredictable behavior on the part of the provider. Witness the following account:

"I went to the hospital at 10 A.M. and gave the hospital permission to collect insurance benefits only. I deliberately did not sign for or give any permission for procedures to be done because my intent was a completely natural childbirth. The doctor had given all indications that this would be so, saying at my first prenatal visit, 'If you wanted heavy medication, I wouldn't want you as a patient.' Regarding any deviation from a natural birth, he said to me, 'We'll have plenty of time to talk about it.'

Student nurses who did not identify themselves, leading me to believe they were staff nurses, came in and probed deep into my abdomen many times to listen to the baby with the fetascope. This probably elicited the note on my hospital record that the patient appeared hostile and refused blood pressure and fetal heart checks. I also refused the IV. At 5:30 my doctor came into the hospital saying only, 'What's the matter? Why don't you want the IV. Scared of needles?' In a threatening tone he asked me if I wanted to go to another hospital. I was stunned. The physical difficulty of leaving at that point put me at a disadvantage, so I was given the IV. I was afraid to refuse, but hoped also that my acquiescence would stem his obvious anger. It didn't. He gave me such a painful internal exam that it felt as though spears were going through me, coupled with explosions in my head. I screamed and then sobbed as he withdrew his hand and wrist covered with blood.

He ordered an epidural and went out to talk to my husband about a Cesarean. The fetal heart was fine. I was dilating, so my husband refused. At seven o'clock, obviously angry, the doctor pulled Scott out with forceps so hard that the nurses held me because I was being pulled off the foot of the table."

Couples who try to touch all the bases in planning their second birth experience may find in the hospital that there are bases still untouched:

"I had a short, tumultuous two-hour labor, and I really needed medication for pain relief. I was amazed to be told that I couldn't have pain medication unless a fetal heart monitor was attached for five minutes first to make sure the drug didn't affect the baby. That's a real switch. I thought the one thing you could count on was an injection of pain-killer whether you wanted it or not! I was never informed of this before I went to the hospital."

Another woman says, "I felt as though I were in a correctional institution, or maybe a mental hospital. I seemed to have no rights at all, including privacy and dignity. They wouldn't even let me leave after the birth unless I left my baby at the hospital. They threatened a court order to keep it because some lab tests said the baby's blood sugar was low—whatever that means. They starved me through a day and a half of intermittent labor. They kept trying to get me to take Maalox. They were angry when I refused to let them induce labor to get on with it. My membranes were broken so I couldn't go home in early labor. The baby got a skin infection there. It is a horrifying memory. I can't let it happen again."

Another woman, a nurse herself, says, "We went to the hospital after several hours of labor, and when I got there I was told I came too soon and to go home. We came back, almost guiltily, an hour later. Contractions were so strong I was worried that I wouldn't make it through natural childbirth. Then I found I was fully dilated. I'd done transition at home."

Still another mother says, "I would have thought a non-stop forty-eight-hour labor to be horrendous and that I would have opted right out of prepared childbirth. Instead, Bob and I worked and struggled. The birth was the easiest part and wonderful. We did it. We can cope with anything now."

As we have seen throughout this book, and will discuss below, there are things that parents can do to help prevent such horror stories.

## CHOOSING AN OBSTETRICIAN OR MIDWIFE, AND THE PLACE OF BIRTH

Some choose the location of birth first and the practitioner second. Others choose the obstetrician first and check the hospital affiliations later. Hospital staff may answer questions about the obstetrician's mode of practice and therefore aid the selection process. Most hospitals offer tours or will even arrange for individual couples to tour the labor and delivery area. Alternative birth centers may also be visited. Input from women's health groups, breast-feeding organizations such as La Leche, and childbirth education associations is generally helpful. Whom do the home-birth people use for backup prenatal, birth, and postpartum care? What are the options within a reasonable distance from home?

Interviewing obstetricians in person generates a charge for the visit. Some screening of obstetricians may be done without charge, however, in a brief phone call. Two or three prepared questions, like those below, about attitude or practice will help you decide whether it is reasonable to schedule a visit.

Specific requests should be brought up early. The hope, usually unfulfilled, may be that the obstetrician will at some time during the pregnancy draw up a chair to talk about his or her perceptions of birth and how it will be handled, the hospital setup, and the respective roles of parent and obstetrician. However, the couple will in almost every case be required to take the initiative. Both parents should attend prenatal visits, especially those that involve discussion. Occasionally, a couple foregoes the exam to have time to talk. During most such visits there is no internal examination, and the checks on blood pressure and urine can be done at another time. In any event, prenatal care is not paid for by the visit. Internal exams are usually done only at the initial visit and at the end of the pregnancy. Couples can schedule more visits if the physicians are willing. An interview may need to be held with every member of a group practice who may possibly be present at delivery, unless one physician will vouch for the others that what is decided will be acceptable to every doctor in the practice.

Whatever aspects in the sequence of childbirth are most important to the individual couple should be discussed first. All may have to be discussed or agreed on before the selection of an obstetrician or midwife is made. A list may be drawn up. "Do you see any problem with any of our plans, provided all is within normal limits? This is the type of birth we are looking for," is the straightforward, non-argumentative approach.

Questions eliciting attitude are useful. "How do you feel about routine episiotomies?" "What do you think of the birthing rooms?" "How do you feel about the increased Cesarean rate?" "Will there be any problem if I refuse the IV?"

Other possible questions are: "How many of your patients

deliver in positions other than lithotomy?" "How many of your deliveries occur with regional anesthesia?" "How many spontaneous?" "How many of your patients breast feed?"

Some of the answers may be checked with hospital record books in which each day's deliveries are recorded—who delivered, the doctor's name, anesthesia if any, whether forceps were used. The number of Cesareans done is also available. Maternity supervisors at the hospital may be contacted for information, and upon request the supervisor may allow prospective patients to leaf through a few pages. Others may also have reason to inspect the records. The book is not so public that the confidentiality of patients may be violated.

Examples of answers to watch out for are: "You're the only one who ever asked that." "It's for your safety." "Don't worry, I only do it when I have to." "You should have faith in your doctor." "We can't take chances." "It's a hospital rule." "You have to think of your baby." Anecdotes of alleged disasters when a woman refused to cooperate with her doctor's advice may be trotted out to substitute for honest discussion. Often parents are placed on the defensive, by having to defend a request which is only ordinary, such as being allowed to walk during labor or having the baby placed on her abdomen after birth.

There are many emotions involved in becoming a parent. If the visit seems uncomfortable, you may want to interview another obstetrician. Going as a couple is preferable to the woman going alone to the prenatal appointments, for several reasons, one of which is that the obstetrician sees them as parents instead of seeing her as one of a roomful of women in the waiting area.

There is no real quality control for prenatal care. Obstetricians are free to prescribe potentially harmful drugs, restrict weight gain, order diuretics, and induce labor.

Always, the parents must remember that the prime responsibility in pregnancy is theirs, to eat well, rest, exercise, avoid drugs that are not absolutely necessary, and to avoid alcohol and tobacco, whether or not their doctor tells them to.

It is good to know your obstetrician's attitudes and practices early, before a final selection is made, but, if necessary, obstetricians can be changed during pregnancy. Parents have even changed obstetricians during labor:

"The night we went into labor we found that our obstetrician had gone on vacation without telling us, leaving a replacement whom we hadn't met. I called an obstetrician whom we had interviewed earlier and liked, but who was quite far away. He said to bring Anne to the hospital and he would check her. So we changed doctors and hospital!"

"We came in too early and hung around a day and a half. My obstetrician wanted to induce me. I have fast labors so I didn't want to go home. We left the hospital. We felt that we were going to have a 'nothing' experience. We went to a midwife in another hospital, when I was already in labor. The experience was fantastic."

The more knowledge couples have, the more input they have into decisions. Misinformation may be given. "We get a better outcome with a Cesarean for breeches," parents may be told. Not only is there no evidence for this, but a Vermont study of 467 breech births showed no improvement in outcome with a Cesarean in terms of either medical problems or deaths.

"You won't feel anything," does not constitute informed consent.

A trustee of a hospital asks at a board meeting, "Why are there so many Cesarean sections now?" and receives the answer, "Patients are not taking their medications, and this prolongs their labors."

Parents may prefer an attitude of watchful expectancy to an obstetrically managed birth. To ensure this, they may select a midwife or bring their own labor-support person with them.

Technology is not a phenomenon of the last few years or even of hospital birth as it came to be in the 1920s. In the nineteenth century balloons were occasionally inserted into the uterus to induce labor, the concept being that a small baby would deliver more easily. Women did not lie down for birth until Louis XIV ordered it so that he could watch his mistresses give birth, and thereby changed a birth custom long before anesthesia was available to immobilize women on their backs.

Physicians' work hours are incredibly long, even with group practice. There isn't time to explain. Physicians may become insulated from the issue of the safety of technology, and only recently is the legal picture changing. Traditionally, physicians have felt more vulnerable if all possible procedures were not done. However, the trend now is in the direction of increased vulnerability for "sins of commission" instead of "sins of omission" only.

Insurers of physicians and hospitals recommend that to reduce vulnerability to malpractice suits, medical-care providers not abandon or neglect a patient without providing access to a qualified substitute, document-informed consent, document refusal, or noncompliance on the part of the patient, keep good records, and never guarantee a cure as a result of treatment. Also, they must remember that consent of parents is required, with few exceptions, for treatment of a minor.

Intervention is not equivalent to prevention. It is not equivalent to care. It is not equivalent to safety.

In regard to patients' rights, situations may become complicated. Even in the following extreme case a patient may not realize that there is such a thing as patients' rights. In fact, the patient is grateful to the hospital.

The following actual incident occurred in 1980 and is described by a hospital nurse in the Boston Association for Childbirth Education newsletter.

SCENE: A greater Boston area hospital which handles over 2,000 births per year. Mrs. Smith's (not her real name) physician suggests that she enter the hospital near the time of her estimated due date so he can induce labor although there is no medical reason for doing so. Even though the FDA has stated that inductions be done only for specific medical reasons, and that the only acceptable method of administering the labor-inducing drug is by intravenous drip, the physician prescribes the tablet form, routinely used at this institution (a lawsuit brought by the manufacturer reversed the FDA's attempts to ban the tablets). The physician leaves the hospital for most of the labor despite the *Physicians' Desk*

*Reference* recommendation that a qualified physician be available at all times during administration of the drug. After the dose exceeds the maximum recommended daily dose by 26 percent, the baby becomes severely distressed. It is apparent that an immediate Cesarean section is necessary. However there is no anesthesiologist available on the premises because they are only available at this hospital from 7 A.M. to 5 P.M. The physician performs the surgery without anesthesia. The baby is saved after vigorous resuscitation measures. Mrs. Smith goes into shock but recovers and is grateful to her physician for saving her baby's life.

What is wrong with this story?

Who could have stopped this chain of events, and at what point?

Who was advocating for the mother? For the baby?

When does one stop taking orders and start taking responsibility?

Can the present medical system be expected to police itself?

Have we been misled into thinking the medical profession maintains an unrealistically high standard of ethics?

What happened to the physicians' motto, First, do no harm?

How effective are our "consumer protection" agencies?

## THE "OPTIMUM BIRTH LETTER"

Medical professionals have described these letters as "manifestos" or seen them more positively as written reminders. They have been used by those planning a home birth with hospital backup in addition to those planning a hospital birth. Copies of the letter are hand-delivered to the obstetrician by the parents-to-be, then sent to the labor and delivery area of the hospital. Sometimes it has seemed wise to include copies for the chiefs of obstetrics, anesthesiology, pediatrics, the nursery, and the hospital administrator. Hospital boards, which have ultimate responsibility for the hospital, are also beginning to be involved. Extra copies of the letter are brought at the time of delivery, in case the originals have been lost in the hospital.

The letter may start:

"On or about (DATE) we expect to give birth at (NAME) hospital to our (first, second, etc.) child. Unless a medical problem should arise, in which case we expect both the problem and any required procedural changes to be discussed with us, we request the following. If any of our plans cannot be carried out at your hospital, we wish to be informed of this ahead of time. We have placed asterisks next to the requests that are most important to us."

If a home or alternative birth center is to be the place of birth, the letter to the backup hospital might begin:

"On or about (DATE) we expect to give birth at home (or birth center) to our (first, second, etc.) child. At this time there is no reason to anticipate any change of plans. However, in case of complications, we would come to (NAME) hospital for assistance. Our requests are as follows:"

(The following list is offered as a guide. Parents may withdraw any of their requests at any time before or during labor.)

1. There will be no routine enema or shaving of pubic hair.

2. No medications will be administered without prior consent of the mother, or in the event of her incapacity, the father. This request excludes none and specifically includes oxytoxics, analgesics, barbiturates, and tranquilizers.

3. The amniotic sac will not be artificially ruptured.

4. No intravenous fluids will be given without prior permission or good medical reason as determined by the parents and the physician in consultation.

5. There will be no electronic fetal monitoring, either internal or external. Frequent listening to the fetal heart is expected. A Doptone may be used if desired. (The Doptone is a device using ultrasound, placed on the abdomen making the fetal heartbeat audible. It can be used selectively and intermittently.)

6. The father and/or other support person (names) will remain throughout labor and birth regardless of circumstances, especially if a problem should arise.

7. The mother will wear her own clothing during birth and afterward. The gown will be short and with short, wide sleeves.

8. The mother will walk during labor and will be assisted by staff in assuming whatever position is most comfortable during labor and birth. She will not be arbitrarily confined to bed during labor.

9. There will be no episiotomy without medical reason. The parents or nursing staff may apply warm, wet cloths or oil to the area around the vagina prior to delivery. The perineum will be supported during delivery, and the mother's legs will not be held excessively wide apart.

10. The parents will be the first to touch the baby's head. The mother will "catch" her own baby. (In one letter from parents expecting twins, the letter specified that the father was to catch the first twin.)

11. The room will be warm and the lights dimmed for the birth. Excessive noise will be avoided.

12. The baby will be immersed in a large (so the limbs can float) tub of warm water within a half hour of birth. Parents will participate as desired.

13. The baby will be placed on the mother's abdomen and gently massaged and caressed after being delivered. A blanket will cover the baby. The baby may be nursed within minutes of birth.

14. The baby will not be routinely suctioned.

15. The cord will not be clamped or cut for at least two minutes unless it must be cut to complete the birth of the baby.

16. Silver nitrate drops in the baby's eyes will be delayed for at least one hour after birth. (An occasional birth letter specifies tetracycline ointment six hours after birth instead of silver nitrate. Because silver nitrate is still usually required by state laws, it is difficult to refuse it, although a waiver may be signed.)

17. The third stage of labor (delivery of the placenta) is not to be rushed but is to proceed at its own pace. The use of oxytoxic drugs and manual removal of the placenta are to be reserved for true medical emergencies.

18. The baby is not to be placed in any warming device.

19. The baby is not to receive routine vitamin K.

20. The baby is not to be washed immediately. Blood and meconium will be gently wiped off.

21. All care of the baby is to take place at the mother's bedside. The baby is not to be taken to the nursery.

22. The baby is not to be given a pacifier or bottles of water or sugar water.

23. In-room sibling visitation will be possible. Our child (name, age) will be visiting in our room as soon after birth as we desire. A support person (name) will bring them and remain with them.

24. Our older child is (name, age) to be present at birth if he (or she) desires. The child has been prepared by (name). (This option is available at a very few hospitals, but at many birth centers.)

25. We plan to leave the hospital within six hours of birth if all members of the family are well.

26. We give (or do not give) permission for students, hospital house staff, or other non-essential personnel to be in the room during labor and birth.

27. Our child, if male, is not to be circumcised.

Cesarean birth requests may include:

1. Spinal or epidural anesthesia will be used if possible. There will be no preoperative medications, especially sedative drugs.

2. The father and another support person will remain with the mother at all times regardless of the circumstances, even if, and especially if, the mother should receive general anesthesia for the birth. The father, at least, will witness the birth.

3. The screen at the mother's chest level, blocking view of birth and the newborn's arrival, will be lowered or removed altogether. Modern technique and parent wishes make this device obsolete.

4. The parents will love and nurse the baby while the incision is being closed.

5. There will be no mandatory period in the nursery. Rooming-

in will be immediate and continuous unless there is a genuine problem with the baby. Parents and baby will be in the recovery room after delivery.

6. There will be no supplemental feedings. Extra breast milk will be given by donors if needed.

## "WHAT HAPPENS IF I SAY NO?" LEGAL RIGHTS

No parent expects to or wants to involve the law in the birth of a child. There are usually better ways of resolving a conflict. Only when communication breaks down totally do legal rights become of concern. Although there is a framework of law, legal decisions in a given situation cannot be predicted perfectly. A brief outline of the framework follows.

Public health regulations were designed at a time when control of epidemics was the primary issue, and therefore a health regulation has stronger impact than regulations in many other areas. The state health departments have codes regarding equipment, space, and some other aspects of care, as well as licensing responsibilities. The federal government is involved in funding programs and checking product safety. Hospitals themselves may promulgate regulations such as those that for so long barred fathers from delivery rooms.

The courts are outcome-oriented. Usually obvious harm must be demonstrated for patients to win a case. Errors are not by themselves grounds for suit, especially if the physician was following the standard care used by his peers, whatever this may be. Action can be brought in such cases as invasion of one's right to bodily or informational privacy, denial of access to records, breach of confidentiality.

A standard text used when discussing this topic is *The Rights of Hospital Patients* by George Annas (Avon Books, 1975).

For childbirth, as with any medical condition, patients may not force a hospital to provide a service. They can only refuse what is offered. A conscious, mentally competent adult may refuse treatment, including even life-sustaining and emergency measures. Mental incompetency may not be inferred from the act of refusal, even in the case of a person in a mental hospital. The refusal may stand even if it is as apparently irrational as the fear of a needle.

Although the patient may refuse any treatment, if a patient consistently refuses to participate in any treatment program, it might be possible for the hospital to ask the patient to leave. The patient would sign a form relieving the hospital of responsibility.

A patient of sound mind may leave the hospital at any time. If the hospital tries to prevent the patient from leaving by threat or physical force, it can be sued for false imprisonment. This is true even if the patient has not paid the bill. Conversely, if a person desires admission to a hospital and an emergency is found to exist, a hospital with emergency facilities is required by law to render the appropriate service. For example, a woman planning a home birth, who requires emergency hospital services, cannot be denied care.

Before treatment is given, the physician must give the patient information about the procedure and its possible risks. This is called informed consent. The concept of informed consent is based on the doctrine of battery, wherein intentionally touching another person without permission, except in an emergency, is a legal wrong. Informed consent, fundamental to traditional medical ethics, means that the patient understands the prospective medical procedures based on adequate information of his or her condition. However, this law is difficult to enforce. Medical records may contain the words "discussed with patient," but if the patient does not sign the form, the patient may disagree later that there was informed consent.

Information given to the patient as a basis for informed consent must be that which a "reasonable man" would need to make a decision. This is called "the reasonable man" test.

In childbirth, there are two patients, as obstetricians frequently remind parents. Parents do not have life-and-death authority over their children. Therefore, the courts may order treatment for children overriding parent refusal. Usually only in extreme cases involving potential death or permanent disability would this be likely to occur.

The American College of Obstetrics and Gynecology, when home birth first became an option, claimed that refusing treatment for the unborn or newborn should constitute child abuse.

Refusal of newborn care or the desire to remove the newborn from the hospital may result in the threat, if not the actuality, of a court order obtained by the hospital to remove the child from parental custody in order to continue hospital care. This has actually occurred.

However, most parents can leave the hospital with their child almost immediately after birth with no difficulty, and home birth, as stated previously, is perfectly legal.

In childbirth there is often uncertainty about what procedures are merely custom, what are opinion, what are written hospital policy. If there is a written policy, who wrote it and why? Who supports it—anesthesiology, pediatrics, obstetrics? Is it in the process of change? Will a hospital staff person sign a statement that a procedure, said to be required, is without risk? Much of obstetrical practice is based more on the "try it, see if it helps" approach than on sound research. Now that pain relief is no longer the highest priority, parents may check the possible drugs that could be used for injection, in the IV or in the regional anesthesia, by perusing the *Physicians' Desk Reference* available in all medical libraries and physicians' offices.

Their personal medical records may be viewed by patients in some states, but not all. Sometimes a physician's presence or other requirements are involved.

When patients become assertive, the physician may include the words "uncooperative" in the medical record, or even "referred to psychiatrist," apparently as a result of refusing treatment. This is partly as a protection against possible future legal problems. Refusals must be noted so that the physician feels more protected by not doing standard procedures. However, this is not a total protection, because the law does not allow the provider of care to waive all responsibility. The knowledge that the patient will review the record may help to prevent excessive unflattering remarks because the physician may not wish to alienate a patient. He is unhappy also if derogatory remarks about the care provided are spread throughout the medical community.

The threat of abandonment by the physician is powerful. However, the patient cannot truly be abandoned without replacement of care in situations of medical need. This applies to physicians and hospitals. On the other hand, the physician does not have to provide a type of care that he or she does not wish to give or deems irresponsible. The patient can sign a waiver, but the physician cannot give all responsibility to the patient, the assumption being that the patient doesn't know the implications of what he or she is doing. But if a procedure is done to parents or their child without prior consent, the case can be one of assault. If parents are not in the newborn nursery or with their hospitalized infants or children, they can hardly give consent for everything done, certainly not informed consent. The consent is taken for granted in many cases.

As stated previously, the general consent form signed on admission is a protection for neither medical-care provider nor patient.

Not only may it be amended before signature, it need not be signed at all. Better protection for all is provided if the patient signs individually for procedures.

Not that refusal of hospital childbirth procedures is inherently desirable. Reasons for using various procedures have been explained, as well as reasons for not. Parents, in cooperation with health professionals, must assess needs and desires. When making decisions about whether to use various tests, whether it be ultrasound, amniocentesis, or electronic monitoring, some couples consider whether or not they will make any changes in what they do as a result of the test results. For example, if the baby is determined to be large for dates or is not moving actively in the uterus, will they have an induced labor? Would the monitor tracing help in making a decision to speed labor with Pitocin? Would it help to determine the need for Cesarean section? Couples, with their medical-care providers decide, too, what other interventions may be required as a result of the procedure; for example, an amniotomy, and consider whether the benefits might outweigh the risks. Amniotomy may increase the risk of cord compression and resulting fetal distress. But if the fetal heart is slowing or becoming irregular, there might be a discussion of breaking the membrane to see if the fluid is stained with meconium. The two factors help to determine possible fetal distress, so the possible resulting speeded labor after amniotomy may in this case be desirable to get the baby delivered soon. If the baby's heart rate has dropped substantially, the decision for a necessary Cesarean may be facilitated by amniotomy if one knows whether the fluid is clear or meconium-stained. No labor is routine. Intelligent on-going observation and assessment are required because routine standing orders for a series of interventions will act to increase the chances of an otherwise unnecessary Cesarean.

The American Hospital Association's "Patient's Bill of Rights" acknowledges that the traditional physician-patient relationship takes on a new dimension when care is rendered within an organizational structure. It states that "no catalog of rights can guarantee for the patient the kind of treatment he has a right to expect. A hospital has many functions to perform, including the prevention and treatment of disease, the education of both health professionals and patients, and the conduct of clinical research." It encourages recognition of the patient's dignity as a human being, the right to considerate and respectful care, and the right to information, including information necessary to give informed consent prior to the start of any procedure or treatment. It recognizes the right of refusal of treatment to the extent permitted by law, the right to information on medical alternatives, and the rights of privacy and confidentiality.

The American College of Obstetrics and Gynecology in association with the American Academy of Pediatrics, the American College of Nurse-Midwives, and the Nurses' Association of ACOG, through the establishment of a task force, launched a major national drive to promote family-centered maternity and newborn care in hospitals.

The task force endorses:

• The option of a birthing room (so that patients will not have to be moved from labor room to delivery room moments before the birth).

• The presence of the husband or another support person throughout birth and afterward to assist in the care of the baby.

• Flexible rooming-in with the goal of maximum desired mother-infant contact, especially during the first 24 hours. If it is necessary to take the infant to the intensive-care nursery, the mother should be allowed to visit and feed the baby.

• Permitting children to visit with the mother and father in a special family room.

- Optional early release from the hospital for mother and baby.
- Breast-feeding if desired. Handling the baby is encouraged immediately after delivery.
- Childbirth classes.

The American College of Obstetrics and Gynecology has made the following general comments in response to a government report attempting to evaluate risks of obstetric practices. "Some problems with technology are acknowledged."

"• ACOG agrees with the overall conclusions that research results are inconclusive regarding the benefit/risk relationship of various obstetric practices and that more organized efforts are needed to help answer questions that remain unresolved. ACOG is willing to work with HEW and other interested parties in trying to resolve the issues.

- It [ACOG] is as, if not more, concerned as critics about the benefits and risks of obstetric practices, and wants to see that (1) obstetric procedures are appropriate, (2) the procedures are used in appropriate circumstances, and (3) the procedures are correctly applied. It acknowledges that some incorrect applications have occurred but believes these have been infrequent.

- Some conclusions about the risks or harmful effects of some obstetric procedures may be unwarranted because adverse consequences that sometimes occurred may have resulted from incorrect or inappropriate use of a procedure, as opposed to an inherent problem with the procedure.

- The professional liability aspect of obstetrics and the importance of professional judgment in determining appropriate procedures to use in individual situations need to be considered in any evaluation of obstetric practices. Obstetrics is one of the highest risk categories in terms of professional malpractice liability. Many obstetricians have switched to other areas because of this. Practicing obstetricians must consider the potential liability aspects of their procedures and the needs of individual patients. Accordingly, obstetrics cannot be practiced in 'cookbook' fashion.

- While ACOG does want to cooperate with organizations . . .

which have responsibilities for regulating or evaluating certain aspects of obstetric procedures, it does not believe that such organizations should dictate patient treatment procedures to physicians.

• It questions the validity and usefulness of findings and conclusions on obstetric practices based on data from the HEW National Institute of Neurological and Communicable Disease Collaborative Study. Major changes have occurred in obstetric practices since the 1959–66 period in which children studied were born. For example, today, high forceps are rarely used and general anesthetics used less frequently. Also, the study's methodology was not appropriate for evaluating obstetric practices.

• It agrees that more public and patient education on childbirth procedures is needed. It does not believe that patient package inserts being considered by FDA are appropriate because they do not and cannot relate the benefits or risks of a particular medication to an individual patient's situation."

Hospitals are in the situation of being oversupplied with technology. These institutions cannot refer their normal patients to a low-technology center because, in order to survive, they need the normal cases as well as the high-risk group. The normals support those with pathology, because without the normals the high-technology centers would not have enough patients to meet their costs. Any disturbance of the delicate equilibrium existing among hospitals, physicians, nurses, medical schools, insurance companies, and commercial supply houses can be seen as a threat. The initial response may be to "blame the patient."

When a problem is perceived, some members of the public and also some providers of medical care will leap to the so-called football analogy of forceful action to solve a problem. If fetal illness is the problem, then more and better technology is the solution.

Protests against the analogy can elicit self-righteous and simplistic accusations. However, other providers are grateful to patients for taking initiatives that they, as professionals working within an institution, may feel unable to do. If patients are legally allowed to take more responsibility, the providers may lose some power, but may also be better protected legally. The trend is for courts to view the physician-patient relationship as a partnership rather than as a monopoly.

For expectant couples and the public in general, birth is knowable. The procedures that have become associated with birth are knowable, as are the forces affecting medical-care providers. With this knowledge, there can be a dialogue between those who give and those who receive childbirth services. Enormous benefits can, and have, accrued to both.

# Glossary

**Amniotomy:** Surgical rupture of the fetal membrane in induction of labor.

**Analgesic:** A medication used during labor to raise the threshold of pain or induce sleep.

**Anesthetic:** A substance introduced into the body to block sensation in one region of the body or to cause loss of consciousness.

**Anterior:** The forward or belly surface of the body.

**Apgar Score:** An evaluation of five factors in the newborn infant at one minute and five minutes after birth: color, pulse, respiration, muscle tone, and reflex irritability.

**Barbiturate:** An analgesic medication to induce sleep.

**Bilirubin:** Yellow bile derived from the metabolism of hemoglobin in red blood cells.

**Bonding:** A process based on the psychological phenomenon of imprinting, occurring most obviously between parents and their young during the period immediately after birth when parents and young first see, touch, hear, and even smell each other; through this contact the mutual attachment process begins.

**Breech:** The infant's position in the uterus in which the baby is buttocks-down instead of the usual head-down position.

**Cephalopelvic Disproportion:** The situation where the baby's head is too large to pass through the mother's pelvis.

**Cervix:** The mouth of the uterus.

**Cesarean Section:** A surgical procedure involving incision through the abdomen and uterus that allows the baby to be removed through the abdomen.

**Childbirth Education:** Includes factual information about the childbirth processes and preparation for participation in the childbirth experience.

**Colostrum:** The yellowish substance produced by the breasts for the baby before the milk comes in.

**Conduction Anesthesia:** A regional block anesthesia such as epidural, spinal, saddle block. It permits consciousness, but interferes with the conduction of sensory nerve impulses to the brain. The anesthetized region depends on where the anesthetic substance is injected.

**Demerol:** A narcotic that raises the pain threshold.

**Diaphragm:** The muscular-membranous partition separating the abdominal and thoracic cavities. It descends when air enters the lungs during inhalation.

**Dilation:** A term referring to the amount of opening (measured in fingers or centimeters) of the cervix during the first stage of labor.

**Dystocia:** Abnormal labor, often used in association with the term "uterine inertia." May be due to the size or position of the fetus or other factors.

**EDC:** The anticipated approximate date of birth, sometimes called the expected date of confinement.

**Effleurage:** The gentle, rhythmic stroking of the abdomen during a contraction which was first used in France.

**Engagement:** Passage of the largest diameter of the infant's head into the pelvic brim. Also called "lightening" or "dropping".

**Epidural:** A conduction anesthesia introduced into the epidural space in the lower back below the level of the spinal cord.

**Episiotomy:** Surgical incision made by the obstetrician just before delivery to enlarge the vaginal opening.

**Family-centered Maternity Care:** Care focused on the importance of family unity and closeness during the days surrounding birth according to the needs and choices of the couple.

**Fetascope:** An instrument similar to a stethoscope for direct listening to the fetal heart during pregnancy and labor.

**First Stage of Labor:** The stage when the cervix dilates while the baby remains in the uterus.

**Forceps:** An instrument for assisting delivery with the basic design of two attached blades, over a foot long, spoon-shaped at the ends to fit over the sides of the infant's head.

**General Anesthesia:** Anesthesia that removes consciousness and therefore removes pain sensations from all parts of the body.

**Gluteal Muscles:** The muscles in the buttocks.

**Induction, Induced Labor:** A labor started by puncture of the membrane around the baby or by giving an oxytoxic drug, or both.

**Labor Support Person:** One who remains with the patient (labor sitting) during labor: a friend or a person hired by the patient, not the hospital.

**Let-down Reflex:** A neurohormonal reflex in which the pituitary gland is stimulated, usually by the sucking of the baby, to secrete oxytocin. The milk sacs then tighten and squeeze milk down to the milk-collecting sinuses.

**Lithotomy Position:** The delivery position in which the mother lies flat on the table with her legs up in stirrups.

**Lochia:** The bloody vaginal discharge from the uterus, similar to a heavy menstrual period, during the first two weeks after birth, gradually turning brown and tapering off during the third week.

**Meconium:** The newborn's intestinal contents formed during pregnancy, a black, tarry substance expelled soon after birth, and sometimes before or during birth.

**Medication:** Analgesic drugs such as barbiturates, narcotics, and tranquilizers that act to relieve pain in the first stage of labor.

**Narcotic:** A drug producing a reversible condition characterized by stupor or insensitivity.

**Natural Childbirth:** The term first used to describe the approach of Grantly Dick-Read, and a term that has aroused as many misconceptions as permissive parenthood. In the past it was used to describe a birth during which no medication or anesthesia was used, whether or not training and education were employed. To some, it can imply a primitive kind of childbirth in which modern knowledge plays no part, or a rigid system of no obstetrical interference regardless of circumstances. At present the term "natural childbirth" is usually used to mean prepared childbirth.

**Nembutol:** A barbiturate which may be used during labor.

**Occiput:** The back part of the baby's head which first presents itself as it crowns just before delivery.

**Oxytocin or Oxytoxic Substance:** The hormone that stimulates the uterus to contract. This is also involved in the let-down reflex during breast-feeding and in other physiological responses.

**Paracervical:** A local anesthesia given by inserting a needle through the vagina into the cervix during the dilation stage of labor.

**Parent Education:** Education of parents at any point in their development as parents with or without the accompanying physical preparation and training for participation in childbirth or factual information about the processes and events of labor, delivery, and breast-feeding.

**Pelvic Floor:** The area between the thighs and between the vagina and rectum.

**Perinatal:** The perinatal period in medical statistics is considered to begin with completion of 28 weeks' gestation and to end 1–4 weeks after birth. Usually the 1-week figure is used.

**Perineum:** The pelvic floor and the associated structures occupying the pelvic outlet. It is bounded in front by the pubic symphysis, in back by the coccyx, and on the sides by the ischial tuberosities (the bones one sits on).

**Pitocin:** A trade name for an oxytoxic substance.

**Placenta:** The embryological organ, often known as the "afterbirth," which attaches to the uterus and taps into the maternal blood supply to filter oxygen and nutrients and remove waste products for the embryo. It also functions as a gland secreting female hormones.

**Placental Transfusion:** The process by which the baby is held lower than the mother's body to allow the remaining blood in the placenta to flow into the cord and into the baby before the cord is cut.

**Posterior Position:** The position in which the occiput, or back part of the baby's head, is toward the mother's back instead of in the usual anterior position.

**Postpartum:** The period of time between the birth and the six-week medical checkup.

**Prepared Childbirth, Participating Childbirth, Educated Childbirth, Cooperative Childbirth:** These terms are used interchangeably, each giving emphasis to an important aspect of the approach. Medication may or may not be used according to individual need and is not defined by any maximum or minimum requirements, but by whether or not the woman knows how to cooperate. Patients awake under conduction anesthesia such as spinals or epidurals, but without preparation for childbirth, are not seen as having prepared childbirth.

**Psychophysical:** A word used to describe any approach to childbirth preparation that uses a combination of psychological and physical techniques to achieve greater comfort, relaxation, and concentration so as to permit participation in childbirth, whether or not analgesia or anesthesia is used.

**Psychoprophylaxis:** Literally, "mind prevention," and more liberally translated, "prevention of pain." An active, directive psychological analgesia aimed at preventing pain and modifying the perception of pain. A physiological basis for its success is also recognized.

**Pudendal Bloc(k):** A regional or conduction anesthesia that anesthetizes the vagina so that the woman does not feel the baby leave her body.

**Saddle Bloc(k):** A conduction anesthesia that numbs the parts of the body that would touch a saddle. It is a "low spinal."

**Seconal:** A barbiturate.

**Second Stage of Labor:** The stage of labor *following* the stage during which the cervix dilates. During the second stage the baby moves down the birth canal.

**Spinal Anesthesia:** A regional anesthesia that temporarily blocks sensation from the lower part of the body and also inhibits the ability to move the legs.

**Spontaneous Delivery:** A delivery in which forceps are not used.

**Toxemia of Pregnancy:** A group of pathologic conditions, essentially metabolic disturbances, manifested by preeclampsia characterized by hypertension, albumin in the urine, and edema (swelling).

**Tranquilizer:** A drug used during the first stage of labor to relieve anxiety and to increase the effectiveness of other drugs, such as the narcotics and barbiturates.

**Transition:** The last part of the first stage of labor, during which the cervix dilates from 7–10 centimeters.

**Trimester:** A three-month span; the first, second, or third three-month period of pregnancy.

**Vernix:** The white, greasy substance that covers the baby's body at birth. It serves to protect the newborn's delicate skin and to facilitate the delivery.

# National and International Organizations Associated with Childbirth

Every state and most communities have childbirth organizations. Although the list is too extensive to give in full, contact with the following organizations will elicit local information on childbirth classes, alternative birth centers, home birth, breast-feeding, midwives, labor support people, hospitals, and obstetricians. This information is usually available for little or no charge.

American Academy of Husband-Coached Childbirth, P.O. 5224, Sherman Oaks, CA 91413.

American Academy of Pediatrics, One Wacker Drive, Chicago, IL 60611.

American College of Nurse-Midwives, 1000 Vermont Avenue, N.W., Washington, D.C. 20005.

American College of Obstetrics and Gynecology, 600 Maryland Avenue, S.W., Washington, D.C. 20024.

American Foundation of Maternal and Child Health, Inc., 30 Beekman Place, New York, NY 10022.

American Public Health Association, 1015 18th Street, N.W., Washington, D.C. 20036.

American Society for Psycho-Prophylaxis in Obstetrics, 1411 K Street, N.W., Washington, D.C. 20005.
    LOCAL GROUPS TEACH LAMAZE, EDUCATIONAL CONFERENCES, LITERATURE.

Association for Childbirth at Home, International, P.O. 39498, Los Angeles, CA 90039.

*Birth and the Family Journal*, 110 El Camino Real, Berkeley, CA 94705.
    CONTAINS ABSTRACTS AND RESEARCH ON BIRTH TOPICS.

Birth and Life Book Store, P.O. 70625, Seattle, WA 98107.
    HAS BOOK AND SUPPLY LISTS, SELLS CHILDBIRTH BOOKS.

Boston Women's Health Collective, P.O. 192, West Somerville, MA 02144.

C-Sec, Inc., 66 Christopher Road, Waltham, MA 02154.
OFFERS CLASSES AND INFORMATION ON CESAREAN BIRTH.

Cascade Birthing Supplies Center, 718 SW 16th Street, Corvallis, OR 97330.

Center for Research on Birth and Human Development, 2340 Ward Street, Suite 105, Berkeley, CA 94705—Lewis Mahl, M.D., Director.

Center for Science in the Public Interest, 1117 Church Street, Washington, D.C. 20036.

Health Research Group, 2000 P Street, N.W., Washington, D.C. 20036.

Home Birth, P.O. 355, Boston University Station, Boston, MA 02215.

Informed Homebirth, P.O. 788, Boulder, CO 80306.

INTACT, P.O. 5, Wilbraham, MA 01095.
PROVIDES INFORMATION ON CIRCUMCISION.

International Childbirth Education Association, P.O. 20048, Minneapolis, MN 55420.
PUBLISHES NEWSLETTER, CONDUCTS CONFERENCES, COORDINATES EFFORTS OF MEMBER CHILDBIRTH EDUCATION GROUPS.

The La Leche League International, 9616 Minneapolis Avenue, Franklin Park, IL 60131.
RESEARCH INFORMATION ON BREAST-FEEDING, LOCAL CHAPTERS, PARENT COUNSELING, GROUP MEETINGS.

Long Island Childbirth Alternatives, P.O. 17, Shoreham, NY 11786.

March of Dimes Birth Defects Foundation, 1275 Mamaroneck Avenue, White Plains, NY 10605.

Maternity Center Association, 48 E. 92nd Street, New York, NY 10028.
HAS INFORMATION ON BIRTH CENTERS AND HAS ITS OWN ALTERNATIVE BIRTH CENTER.

National Association of Parents and Professionals for Safe Alternatives in Childbirth, Inc., Marble Hill, MO 63764.
HAS INFORMATION ON OUT-OF-HOSPITAL AND HOME BIRTH; SPONSORS EDUCATIONAL CONFERENCES.

"The National Institutes of Health, Consensus Development Task Force Report," Office of Research Reporting, Building 31, Room 2432, NICHD, (National Institute for Child Health and Development), 9000 Rockville Pike, Bethesda, MD 20205.

National Midwives Association, P.O. Box 163, Princeton, NJ 08540.

National Women's Health Network, 2025 I Street, N.W., Suite 105, Washington, D.C. 20006.

U. S. General Accounting Office Distribution Section, Room 1518, 441 6th Street, N.W., Washington, D.C. 20548.

> REPORTS TO THE CONGRESS OF THE UNITED STATES. PUBLISHES "EVALUATIVE BENEFITS AND RISKS OF OBSTETRIC PRACTICES— MORE COORDINATED FEDERAL AND PRIVATE EFFORTS NEEDED," HRD-79-85, SEPTEMBER 24, 1979.

# Index